# Defeat Wheat

## Your Guide to Eliminating Gluten and Losing Weight

## By Brian Gansmann

# Also Released by Sakura Publishing

*Touretties*
*Lost Evidents*
*Fortino*
*When Heaven Calls*
*Dump Your Problems!*
*The Legend of Willow Springs Farm*
*Stricken Yet Crowned*
*Did I Really Do My Hair For This?*

# Defeat Wheat

## Your Guide to Eliminating Gluten and Losing Weight

### By Brian Gansmann

ISBN-10    0615522831
ISBN-13    9780615522838

# Disclaimer

This publication is intended to provide helpful and informative material. It is not intended to diagnose, treat, cure, or prevent any health problem or condition, nor is it intended to replace the advice of a physician. No action should be taken solely on the contents of this book. Always consult your physician or qualified healthcare professional on any matters regarding your health and before using any suggestions in this book or drawing inferences from it.

The author and publisher specifically disclaim all responsibility for any liability, loss or risk, personal or otherwise, which is incurred as a consequence, directly or indirectly, from the use of applications of any contents of this book.

Any and all product names referenced within this book are the trademarks of their respective owners. None of these owners have sponsored, authorized, endorsed, or approved this book. Always read all information provided by the manufacturers' product labels before using their products. The author and publisher are not responsible for claims made by manufacturers. The statements made in this book have not been evaluated by the Food and Drug Administration.

# About the Author

Brian's love of food began at a very young age, as his parents owned several restaurants and recently celebrated their 26th anniversary in business. He grew up learning to prepare, know, and love not just ordinary food, but *great* food. In fact, it was this early passion for wholesome cuisine that led him into the retail advertising industry. In 2008, Brian, his business partner, and a Swiss-born chef (who is a member of the American Culinary Federation) founded a successful brokerage firm that creates new items for a number of national retailers and shopping clubs. You may have even seen Brian on NBC, FOX, CBS, ABC, and QVC talking about the benefits of adopting an all-natural diet. His advertising tenure has also included working with the following companies: The Kroger Company, Robert Mondavi Wines, Idaho Potatoes, Hillshire Farms, Red Lobster, Sam's Club, and other well known food/beverage brands.

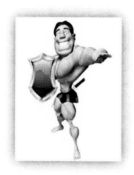

Sometime over the course of working with these companies, Brian was appointed the Director of Marketing for Cedarlane Natural Foods, the second largest frozen organic food company in the nation. While at the helm of Cedarlane, he sold the first "made-with-organic" frozen line that Wal-Mart ever carried. Additionally, he worked one-on-one with Dr. Barry Sears, the author of the New York Times Best Selling Book *The Zone Diet*. The Cedarlane Team and Dr. Sears advanced the development and launch of the Zone Diet frozen meals. These meals adhered to the rigorous standards set forth by Dr. Barry Sears in *The Zone Diet* and other books that he has written over the years. Brian eventually became the spokesperson for the entire Zone Diet frozen line, appearing with Dr. Barry Sears on several national and local mediums.

Today, Brian lives in Denver, Colorado, with his lifelong partner. They have celebrated being together for over sixteen years. They are also the proud owners of two adopted dogs, Weimer, a Weimaraner, and Zoe, a Dalmatian.

# Table of Contents

## Foreword
## By Robin Kline

Nothing Brian undertakes and achieves surprises me. Having known and worked with him for almost 20 years, I have been witness to, inspired by, the beneficiary of, and, ultimately, in awe of Brian's passion—for life writ large, laughter, truth, and always seeking out a better way.

In suffering debilitating symptoms, discovering his intolerance for gluten, and being diagnosed with Celiac disease, Brian brings his razor focus to creating a new life for himself. And, since it's Brian's life, it is brimming with infectious energy, compassion, and upbeat good cheer.

As a registered dietitian, I applaud Brian's dietary choices and his recommended daily eating plan. Both science and Brian's testimony support the tempting menus he introduces. Enjoying small meals throughout the day is an approach many of us can embrace.

As a food lover and culinary professional, I am pleased that Brian focuses on an extremely satisfied palate in this eating-for-life scheme. His love of big flavors, experience in the kitchen, and understanding the demands of 21st Century lives inspire his appealing menu suggestions.

Something compelled you to pick up this book. Maybe you're suffering similar symptoms, fighting lack of energy and intestinal distress, looking for answers. Perhaps you're curious about how one man can turn his life around one step at a time. Or, you simply enjoy good stories about a warrior's journey.

Always engaging, entertaining, and enlightening, *Defeat Wheat* offers ideas, answers, and a potential path to renewed life for many readers.

Robin Kline, MS, RD, CCP
Savvy Food Communications
September 2011

# The Curse of the Ancient Pyramid

I remember the first time I saw the food pyramid in grade school. My teacher clearly pointed out that the biggest portion of the pyramid had all of those colorful wheat-based illustrations. It seemed like all of the pyramid's cartoon-like characters had smiles from ear to ear: a grinning waffle, a happy loaf of bread, a chuckling muffin, and even a box of cereal that was so ecstatic flakes were bursting out of the top of the box like a volcano. However, as I looked at the illustration, I believed that this was some kind of ancient pharaoh diet based on eating loads and loads of wheat with every meal.

After my teacher's lecture about the pyramid, I went home and told my parents that I needed to eat more cereal, more bread, more pasta, more pretzels, more bagels, and more muffins. They listened to me. From that point on, my breakfasts, lunches, snacks, and dinners were rarely prepared without some type of wheat. And for millions of Americans like me, that constant ingestion of wheat catches up with you and eventually the "Curse of the Ancient Pyramid" can bring your life to a screeching halt...

# Chapter One

## The Day That Changed My Life

It was 2008. I had just arrived in Germany on vacation and had picked up a Rick Steves travel book somewhere between Denver International Airport and Munich Airport. I perused the pages of this book, and in case you don't know anything about Rick Steves he prides himself on being able to tour any country on a shoestring budget. Hence, I got the idea of doing a walking tour in Germany. It sounded great at the time, so I proceeded to go on my trek all across the Deutschland.

It was during my visit to Munich, which had been the first city on the walking tour, when something happened that would change my life forever:

I was shot.

Well, not exactly, but that's what it felt like. I suddenly found myself on the ground in the fetal position as a result of a severe abdominal cramp. Everything went gray. I couldn't hear the concerned cries of people that stood around me wondering what had happened. I wondered along with them while clawing at my abdomen in a vain attempt to dig out the pain.

Perhaps Munich's historic pavement, which had seen both world wars, had made me think it was a gunshot wound. I managed to check myself for bullet holes, but there weren't any to be found. Still, I wasn't able to catch my breath or resume a full upright position. All I could do was stare up at the cloud of agony that hung over me.

It was then that, for some reason, I recalled how I had been going to the restroom at least 25 times a day over the past couple of years. I also thought about the conversations that I was having with my doctor for the past year. There *had* to be something in my daily diet that was making me constantly end up on a toilet every five seconds! Furthermore, those trips to the bathroom were almost always accompanied by horrible pains and bloating, much like the abdominal cramp I had just felt that made me face-plant into the ground. But was it something I ate?

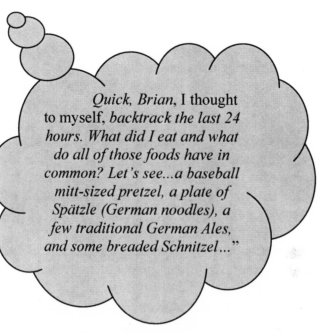

*Quick, Brian,* I thought to myself, *backtrack the last 24 hours. What did I eat and what do all of those foods have in common? Let's see...a baseball mitt-sized pretzel, a plate of Spätzle (German noodles), a few traditional German Ales, and some breaded Schnitzel...”*

"Oh my God," I murmured. My painstaking scowl slowly turned into an accomplished grin. "It's the wheat that's been doing this to me for the past few years. How could I not have figured this out earlier?"

Ladies and gentlemen: I had almost been assassinated by bread.

Upon returning to the States, I was officially diagnosed with Celiac disease by my primary physician. Celiac disease is also known as "gluten intolerance", and the latest statistic is that it affects 1 in 133 Americans. Yet, out of these 2,131,019 people, 97% of them are estimated to not be diagnosed with Celiac disease.[1] I suppose this makes it easy to understand why I overlooked the condition as being one of the possible reasons for my pain and suffering. Upon closer inspection

---

[1] "1 in 133 have Celiac Disease", February 10, 2003 edition of *Archives of Internal Medicine.*

of this autoimmune disorder, I discovered that it can have a variety of adverse affects on the human body: chronic diarrhea, fatigue, malnutrition, abdominal bloating, and failure to thrive (in children). Celiac disease is caused by the body's reaction with gluten, a glycoprotein that is found primarily in wheat, as well as barley and rye. When a celiac's digestive tract is exposed to gluten, the immune system cross-reacts with the small bowel tissue and creates a highly inflammatory environment, nearly wiping out the small hair-like lining in the small intestines called the "villi". These are also known as "villous atrophy" and are the primary tools that our bodies use to absorb nutrients into the blood. Without villi, the body is severely handicapped in its ability to absorb nutrients and vitamins. Hence, the fatigue and malnutrition sets in when your body doesn't receive its daily nourishment.

While there are some similarities to a celiac reaction to protein, it is not the same thing as having a wheat allergy. As you will find out later in this book, trying to pinpoint the cause of all the initial symptoms was a very difficult feat for me. If you are in fact an undiagnosed celiac and you continue to eat wheat, you will increase your chances of gastrointestinal cancer by a factor of 40-100 times that over the normal population, according to *The American Journal of Gastroenterology*.[2] No medication exists that will stop the internal bodily combat when gluten interacts with the body. The only effective treatment for celiac disease is to follow a strict 100% gluten-free diet.

A person diagnosed with Celiac disease also must rely on their eyes and read every label on every food package. Becoming vigilant at the grocery store takes time, though. There are many items that contain gluten that are completely unlabeled, and some foods even omit gluten

---

[2] "40-100 Times more chances of gastrointestinal cancer", Coeliac disease and lymphoma, *European Journal of Gastroenterology and Hepatology*, 2006 18:131-2. Kumar, Parveen -Revolution Health.

from their list of ingredients! Take it from me, I've had to learn about this the hard way, but I promise to help you avoid my pitfalls and show you ways to avoid making stomach-busting mistakes using my practical, everyday guidelines for avoiding gluten.

## I Don't Have a Problem with Gluten, so Why Should I Listen to Your Advice?

I knew that eliminating wheat and gluten from my diet would make me feel 1000% better. What I *didn't* know was that it would also make me stronger, more alert, more satiated, and leaner than ever before! It was like my muscles that had grown dormant with age suddenly became alive. I even became reacquainted with abdominal muscles that I hadn't seen since swimming competitively in high school, and I'm in my forties!

My perspective on life changed, as well. You see, I don't view Celiac disease as a problem for me. It's actually been a fantastic opportunity to share with everyone I meet the benefits of living a gluten-free lifestyle. I want to tell every single person who is ingesting too much wheat and gluten that this could be you: toned, lean, and making healthier food selections at the grocery store that are devoid of complaining groans and a better-than –the-rest pretense! I'm selling you a chance to be happy by learning to not just eat right, but to live right, too.

Hopefully, by the end of reading this book and regardless of your condition, you will be able to do all of the following, just by eliminating or reducing wheat and gluten from your diet:

- ✓ Lose weight
- ✓ Get reacquainted with your hidden abdominal muscles
- ✓ Increase overall strength and stamina
- ✓ Maximize the benefits of working out
- ✓ Maintain emotional well-being and peak mental alertness
- ✓ Combat the effects of aging
- ✓ Decrease the recovery time after cardio and weight-lifting
- ✓ ...and turn the heads of your friends, family, associates, and potential partners!

Yes people, YOU can achieve all this and more with a gluten-free diet. Let me show you how!

*Remember:*

*You might have a gluten intolerance and not even be aware of it.*

*Maybe I can even save anyone diagnosed with Celiac disease from having an embarrassing trans-continental celiac moment like I did!*

# Chapter Two

## What's Your Secret?

D o you remember the kid in grade school that would ask the teacher a question and get an answer that didn't quite satisfy his inquisitiveness? It was followed up with, "Why this?", or, "Why that?", or just, "Why?" about another four times. That student was me. Back then, I asked simple questions like, "How does a thermos know to keep a beverage hot or cold?", or, "How does a seed know which way is up if it's buried underneath soil?" I have been asking questions ever since, but now my questions are about complex things—for instance, the functions of the human body.

Now, I'm not a doctor, nor have I ever played one on TV, but I have been blessed to be surrounded by doctors and other health professionals who have explained to me all about the human body in simple layman terms. I learned the answers to my questions thanks to the help of so many people I knew in healthcare, but my "why, why, why?" attitude drove me to look for even more answers on my own:

✓ Why was I feeling so bloated?
✓ What happened to all of my energy?
✓ Why can't I concentrate?
✓ Why do I have all of these embarrassing moments, in and out of the restroom?
✓ Why am I getting a band of fat over my abdomen if I am eating so many supposed "whole grain" foods?
✓ Why all of the lackluster work-outs lately?
✓ Why does my skin look so unhealthy?
✓ Why does my general practitioner want me to visit an internal surgeon?

I went to the book store and bought nearly every book that pertained to Celiac disease. Most of the reading was very technical and scientific, but it was clear that there was a full-blown war between my digestive system and gluten. Wheat had put me through so much misery, but I could have avoided it all if I had just known about gluten's potential for destruction.

However, I will be the first to tell you that what goes around comes around. Perhaps this was Karma's way of paying me back for not fully understanding Celiac disease.

After years of working in the food advertising industry, I was blessed to have received a job as the Director of Marketing for Cedarlane, an all-natural frozen food manufacturer in California. It's not often that someone in his mid-thirties is given the opportunity to become Director of Marketing for the nation's second largest frozen organic food company, but I wasn't going to argue. I took the job without hesitation.

One fact that I quickly learned about manufacturing was that every employee had to wear a variety of hats. Early mornings were typically spent working with food scientists and nutritionists, late mornings with the finance departments, and lunchtime with the sales department. Mid-afternoon until the end of the day I handled all of the customer service issues, questions, or complaints. I called anyone who left a phone number or voice mail and listened to their concerns.

Now, I'll admit that I had absolutely NO idea what a celiac was when I started working there (I began working there right before being diagnosed with the disease). Whenever customers I talked to questioned which of our items contained wheat and which ones didn't, I figured they were oversensitive and being overly cautious about their food choices—especially when I talked to customers that called themselves "celiacs." I was so uneducated about wheat that I nearly lumped these individuals into the same group as vegetarians and vegans!

This was all happening at the time that YouTube was making its debut on the internet and becoming more and more popular as a website. In order to educate myself about what I kept hearing from customers, I went to YouTube and browsed through videos on Celiac disease. One particular five minute animated segment stunned me and certainly changed my perception forever.

Do you remember the closing scene in *Star Wars* when the rebel tie fighters flew down an enormously long corridor to blow up the behemoth Death Star? Laser shots were being fired, lives were being lost, and explosive mayhem existed around every crevasse. Well, that's basically how the celiac story was described in the YouTube video. Instead of the narrow corridor on the perimeter of the Death Star, it was an illustration of a human intestine and the villi (the tiny, hair-like projections in the intestinal walls that absorb vitamins, minerals, and other nutrients) being attacked. It depicted a full-fledged battle being waged inside millions of bodies around the world. The cartoon-like clip also made the battle between the rebels and the empire look docile. In reality, the body rejects gluten as if it were poison. It causes white blood cells to attack the gluten. Somewhat ironic that Darth Vader's storm troopers were all dressed in white and seeing the rebels as poison to the Death Star!

Suddenly, I had a whole new attitude toward the people who called my office, left voice mails, and sent emails about the wheat-based items in our all natural frozen food department. I actually took the time to ask people about their history with Celiac disease and how they feel nowadays without ingesting any type of wheat. Most of these people sounded pretty chipper and full of energy on the other side of the phone.

Their enthusiasm made me want to take this gluten crusade on myself. I started by listening and asking questions. As the Greek Philosopher Epictetus said long ago:

**We have two ears and one mouth so that we can listen twice as much as we speak.**

My willingness to listen helped me hear from others what I had been telling myself all along: gluten was my Death Star.

During my initial attempt to understand celiac disease, I discovered dozens of books that thoroughly detailed the body's inability to absorb nutrients into the bloodstream. I was happy to finally be able to comprehend what was going on inside my body, but the fact that I spent hundreds of dollars on vitamins, nutritional supplements, and pharmacy grade protein powders over the years before knowing this infuriated me! All of those shakes and capsules went on a non-stop, high speed train from my mouth to the toilet bowl and provided no nutritional benefit to my body whatsoever. Despite this, I came to view the revelation about my digestive inadequacies as an opportunity.

First, I had to stop eating wheat. Abolishing wheat from my diet was difficult, but I eventually eradicated any trace of wheat from all my meals. That's when the fun started! I soon found that my shirts were no longer fitting my ever-widening shoulders. I had to pull my belt one extra notch to keep my pants from falling. My cuffs on my short sleeve t-shirts felt tighter over my biceps, many of my clothes had to be given to charity because they didn't fit anymore, and, best of all, I was re-acquainted with my abdomen muscles that I hadn't seen since the days that I swam competitively in high school!

This new wheat-free lifestyle was working in my favor, and I heard comments over and over again like the following:

> ❖ "Hey, what's your work-out look like?"
> ❖ "How did you get so *lean*?"
> ❖ "What does your diet look like?"
> ❖ "How do you keep your skin *looking so good*?"
> ❖ "Why do you always seem to have so much energy?"
> ❖ "How do you get *abs like that*?"
> ❖ "Are you always on top of your game like that in a business meeting?"

With all of these positive questions being posed about my physique and overall well being, it was very obvious that responding aggressively to Celiac disease and listening to opinions and suggestions from my health care friends was working. I didn't have to worry anymore about not having control of my life. I regained control and still have it to this day. The amazing part is that I did all of this by changing my eating habits and adapting a healthy lifestyle.

That's it.

There are no complicated ratios to calculate, no expensive overnight food deliveries to pay for, and no daily points to count. In reality, it's just sensible eating and snacking throughout the day and unlike any other lifestyle/fitness program, you're actually going to have a good time following it. Defeat wheat, and you'll soon be on your way to a body like you've never seen before.

# Chapter Three

## Ruffling Feathers in the Food Industry

A s I've stated before, I was extremely fortunate to have worked on the advertising team that helped invent the slogan: "Pork. The Other White Meat®." Many people seem to laugh when they read those five words together, but the phrase was part of a Harvard case study that clearly demonstrates how our agency and client, The National Pork Board, completely repositioned an entire industry in the minds of the American public.[3] To this day, that slogan has one of the highest unaided awareness levels of any branded or industry campaign.

In fact, a 1988 tracking study conducted by Omaha-based Rozmarin & Associates, Inc., showed that consumers' unaided association of pork as a white meat increased 163% in markets exposed to "White Meat" television ads. Consumer recall of the primary message of the campaign—that pork is a white meat—was as high as 72 % in cities that received an enhanced level of television exposure to the campaign as well.[4]

If you are not familiar with how pork or milk companies operate, they are typically funded from a check-off fund that farmers collect from the entire group in their respective agricultural field. Money is then used to finance the operational expenses related to the promotion of their goods. The larger the industry, the more massive the entire budget devoted toward advertising. For example, you are all familiar with how the Florida citrus companies have told you to drink more orange juice, the cotton industry has told you about the "fabric of our lives", and the dairy industry has made you reminisce about your juvenile days of drinking milk with a silly white moustache. It's all thanks to this check-off fund.

---

[3] Dougherty, Philip H. "ADVERTISING; Dressing Pork for Success", *The New York Times*, January 15, 1987.
[4] "Tracking Study shows porks ads effective", Rozmarin & Associates, Inc., April 1988.

Before the "Pork. The Other White Meat®" campaign launched, there were two goliaths that the pork board had to go up against: the branded poultry industry and the beef industry. Boy, did we have an uphill battle. More and more retailers and food service operators were touting chicken breasts as the gold standard in terms of the healthiest meat while citing studies from renowned dieticians and nutritionists. Poultry was also infiltrating the usual eating incidences that pork owned for centuries: breakfast and lunch. Each week, there was a new turkey bacon or chicken sausage that gave consumers more options in the morning and midday. And even though the ham sandwich had been a favorite pastime in brown bag lunches, new poultry lunchmeats and breast sandwiches were slugging it out for control of the collective American stomach.

While pork's market share was constantly under attack during lunch and breakfast, the beef industry fought to be the main meal choice consumed in the evening. They spent a tremendous amount of money telling us, "Beef: It's What's For Dinner®." Consequently, beef companies exponentially outspent the pork industry on the airwaves and in print.

When you are up against a very "beefy" advertising budget and the wave of positive information regarding boneless chicken, how can you be heard? All you can do is compete in an honest fashion, and that is exactly what we did at my advertising agency. We simply stated pork's case against the behemoths in the meat industry and ended up really ruffling some feathers (pun intended)!

It wasn't too long before press releases started to hit the wire stating our proposed facts:

Pork was on par with a boneless skinless chicken breast in terms of fat, calories, and cholesterol.

Pork was a versatile meat for nearly any time of the day.

While providing a greater amount of vitamins and minerals, many cuts of pork are as lean or leaner than certain cuts of chicken.

Pork tenderloin is just as lean as skinless chicken breast and even meets the government's guidelines for "extra lean."

More and more chefs and food service operators were putting pork onto their white table cloth menus than ever before.

Various medical personnel were recommending certain cuts of pork for a low fat diet.

Pork is economical, easy to prepare, and even easier to carve for a large gathering.

Pork is the most popular meat in the world (in terms of overall tonnage).

Our competitors didn't respond well to our nonchalant strategy of informing the general public with these facts or to us blanketing airwaves everywhere with our slogan. (Say it again with me: "Pork. The Other White Meat®!") We asked people to use their heads when thinking about their daily diet, not their emotions. It worked beautifully for us.

This is where I would like to start with helping you to make a choice about the role of gluten in your diet. Like the poultry advertisements told us in an emotional fashion why you never should sway from their tradition, the facts about wheat may make you think about different combinations of food that simply make more sense.

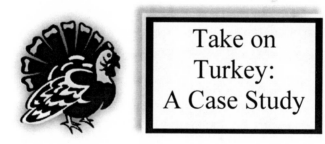

# Take on Turkey: A Case Study

Before we challenge the perception about wheat, I want to leave you with a case study that further illustrates how being informed helped the pork industry win a victory against poultry producers.

When was the last time that you actually cooked a whole turkey? You probably remember going to the store and needing both hands to get the darn thing out of the coffin cooler and into your cart! Then, you brought it home and let it thaw… for a few days. I can remember growing up and seeing the bird defrosting in the sink, on the counter, and even once on the washing machine. When it was time to cook it, you spent another hour just preparing the turkey for its several hundred minutes baking in the oven. "Don't forget to baste it every so often and keep it moist," said the Butterball 800 number.

Once it was finally out of the oven, every family hoped that a relative would arrive on Thanksgiving Day who was a board certified surgeon and could cut around all of the bones on the carcass. This person needed to slice it quick too, as the breast meat easily turned into a slab of turkey jerky with just a few minutes of exposure to the atmosphere. Consequently, all that remained at the end of dinner were dry pieces of turkey.

Thanksgiving is supposed to be a time of getting together with friends and family around an enormous holiday spread, peppered with greenish-orange decorations that make you think of autumn breezes. But, let's face it: Thanksgiving is the "on-deck" position for stress during the fourth quarter holidays. Between the travel, the chaos at the supermarkets, and the overall stress of preparing a perfect meal, you are setting yourself up for a massively imperfect dining experience.

While exchanging stories about the emotions surrounding Thanksgiving Day, our public relations group at Bozell Worldwide (the agency I worked at) came up with a brilliant idea. With just a small amount of research, one of the interns actually discovered that meat and game were typically served at the original Thanksgiving dinner by the colonists—not turkey.[5] Several of our team members were involved in demonstrating the ease of prepping a whole pork loin and baking it in less than an hour. The result was a moist, easy-to-carve, flavorful roast that was right on par with chicken. And, it was even easier to carve for dozens of people at a time while remaining moist and juicy. We

---

[5] Winslow, Edward. "Primary Sources for "The First Thanksgiving" at Plymouth". *Mourt's Relation*. Pilgrim Hall Museum.

didn't need the recorded message from Butterball to tell us about the benefits of basting anymore.

Furthermore, pork was typically purchased fresh so there was no need to defrost it on any of your household appliances. It's considered whole muscle, which means you don't have to clean its internal cavity or solicit help from a medically-inclined relative. There was no need to stand over the oven for hours at a time making sure that the turkey didn't dry out. You could carve a roasted whole loin in front of your guests in *less than 3 minutes.*

The facts were there to "Take on Turkey." Therefore, the team developed a number of press materials with empirical data to substantiate our recommendations for pork rather than turkey at Thanksgiving. The good news was that we received accolades from consumers who related to the stress that surrounds the baking of a bird, not to mention dissecting the bones from the meat. Food editors liked the fact that they could recommend new variations for their readers that enabled the cooks to spend more time with loved ones rather than battling a turkey for several days in the kitchen. And, chefs were happy to offer a variety of Thanksgiving loins to their menus.

The bad news was that the turkey industry thought we were personally attempting to kill a family tradition. While reading their retaliation press release, you could almost hear the keys being punched like the heads of a Whack-A-Mole gaming machine with an oversized padded mallet! How dare we take on a Thanksgiving tradition that the self-proclaiming turkey industry "owns" (although interestingly enough, turkey wasn't officially designated the center of the plate item until the Lincoln administration)!

Regardless, we stuck to our ideology and it appeared that more and more people began to think about the benefits of pork during and beyond Thanksgiving. We turned around a declining industry by simply stating the benefits of looking at a situation in a different way.

Mark Williams, Bozell Worldwide's Vice President & Account Supervisor during the launch of the pork campaign, said:

> **Pork is indeed hot. It's the darling of hot chefs everywhere. You can't go to a great restaurant that doesn't have a pork chop, or pork belly. Bacon has never been hotter, BBQ is everywhere...In the end, the idea that pork is not chicken or beef is really kicking in. It is the perfect alternative...not so much for its porkiness, [but] rather as a result of its versatility...All of this has helped to drive very strong pork demand. Pork prices as about as high as they have ever been in history.**

An anonymous executive from the beef industry made a statement following this revolutionary change that was almost a perfect compliment:

> "The pork people beat us, and with a lot less money."

We didn't need enormous advertising budgets to build our case, just our brains.

As I try to get you to think about your own wheat consumption on a daily basis, I'm going to be making a number of educated recommendations based on data, facts, and personal experiences. Since writing this book, I have already ruffled the feathers of many advocates in the world's gluten-based industries, much like I did with the beef advertising executives. That's okay. The people in charge of the gluten industry have a job to do and that's to increase the world's consumption of wheat. My job is to take a chisel to the ancient food pyramid and carve out a new and improved gluten-free dietary triangle!

# Chapter Four

## The Preliminary Diagnosis

Nowadays, I have to sit down at a restaurant and say to the server: "Now, I'm going to be needy. Do you know if that entrée has any wheat or gluten in it?" The reply is almost always one of bewilderment: "Uh…let me check with the kitchen." When they return to the table (hopefully with the correct information), the server will usually tell me that the item is fine for me to eat, followed by the server elaborating about how more and more patrons are requesting information regarding gluten-free foods. A few of the servers may even mention how it's becoming a big thing. Every single time though, I get this look like they want to know why I can't eat wheat, but they are afraid to come straight out and ask.

I usually bite my tongue whenever a server actually does ask about my need to avoid gluten. Describing the sordid details about a celiac's bowels, especially at a fine eating establishment, doesn't go over well. Along with this, I'm sure they might be thinking that the mere sight of multi-grain toast will make me put my forearm over my eyes like a vampire prostrate before a cross. Or, that my eating a spoonful of Wheaties will engulf me in flames like a vampire in the midday sun.

Guess what folks, I actually *can* eat wheat without spontaneously combusting, but once I've ingested wheat into my stomach, my body has only one objective: to flush the gluten out of my system as quickly as possible. If left inside me, it takes about thirteen hours to create a maelstrom in my stomach and I invariably end up doing the celiac-dash to the nearest bathroom, with pain and embarrassment following close behind me. The whole thing is so unpleasant that I am surprised I lived with the condition for so long and didn't press harder for the truth about my condition. It took collapsing on a cobblestone street in Munich to finally discover what was wrong with me. Thank God it wasn't too late to change.

I'm not alone in thinking this way either. Apparently being a celiac meant sharing the company of some very famous people in the world! The following individuals all had to readjust their lives thanks to their gluten intolerance issues, but obviously their need for change didn't stop any of them from still being successful individuals:

✓ Keith Olbermann (*Countdown with Keith Olbermann*)
✓ Elizabeth Hasselbeck (*The View*)
✓ Heidi Collins (CNN anchor)
✓ Jane Swift (Massachusetts Lieutenant Governor)
✓ Katherine, Duchess of Kent
✓ Susie Essman (*Curb Your Enthusiasm*)
✓ Mickey Redmon (former pro hockey player, does hockey commentary for *Fox Sports Detroit*)
✓ Sarah Vowell (Often heard on NPR radio, she did a funny take on having a wheat allergy and was part of *Living Without* magazine on NPR. She also was "Violet" in *The Incredibles*)
✓ Jennifer Esposito
✓ Thom Hartmann (*Air America Radio*)
✓ Amy Yoder Begley (Competed in Beijing Olympics as a runner)
✓ Cedric Benson (NFL running back for the Cincinnati Bengals—formerly of the Chicago Bears and Texas Longhorns)
✓ Joe Stanton (Cartoonist who draws Batman, Green Lantern, Archie, and Scooby-Do)

So, not only do these amazing and talented people have Celiac disease, it seems that gluten intolerance is something *many* ordinary people have, too. According to the "1 in 133" website here are the comparisons between Celiac disease and other devastating illnesses:[6]

| Illness | Number of American Sufferers: |
|---|---|
| Gluten Sensitivity | <u>18 million Americans (Alessio Fasano, 2011)</u> |
| Celiac Disease | at least 3 million Americans |
| Autism | 556,000 Americans |
| Crohn's Disease | 500,000 Americans |
| Cystic Fibrosis | 30,000 Americans |
| Down Syndrome | 350,000 Americans (42,000 of those diagnosed also have Celiac disease) |
| Epilepsy | 2.7 million Americans |
| Hemophilia | 17,000 Americans |
| Infertility (unexplained) | 610,000 American women (36,600 of those also have Celiac disease) |
| Lupus | 1.5 million Americans |
| Multiple Sclerosis | 400,000 Americans |
| Parkinson's Disease | 1 million Americans |
| Rheumatoid Arthritis | 2.1 million Americans |
| Type 1 Diabetes | 3 million Americans (180,000 of those diagnosed also have Celiac disease) |
| Ulcerative Colitis | 500,000 Americans |

---

[6] Table retrieved from http://www.1in133.org/info/#how.

As you can see, gluten intolerance is widespread in America. Perhaps it's important then to take a closer look at some very sobering statistics on what this means for me and you. According to the National Foundation for Celiac Awareness, here are some of the most staggering facts about Celiac disease:

✓ Celiac disease is an autoimmune digestive disease that damages the villi of the small intestine and interferes with absorption of nutrients from food.
✓ An estimated 3 million Americans across all races, ages, and both genders suffer from Celiac disease.
✓ 95% of celiacs are undiagnosed or misdiagnosed with other conditions.[7]
✓ 6-10 years is the average time a person waits to be correctly diagnosed.[8]
✓ 5-22% of celiac patients have an immediate family member (1st degree relative) who also has Celiac disease.
✓ Celiac disease can lead to a number of other disorders including infertility, reduced bone density, neurological disorders, some cancers, and other autoimmune diseases.
✓ $5,000-$12,000 is the average cost of misdiagnosis per person/per year of Celiac disease, not including lost work time.
✓ There are NO pharmaceutical cures for Celiac disease.

---

[7] Fasano, A., et al. *Arch Intern Med.* 2003;*163*:286-292.
[8] Leffler, Daniel, MD, MS, The Celiac Center at Beth Israel Deaconess Medical Center.

- ✓ A 100% gluten-free diet is the only existing treatment for celiacs today.
- ✓ A positive attitude, 100% of the time, helps celiacs create a gluten-free lifestyle for themselves and their affected family members.
- ✓ The Celiac disease diagnosis rate may reach 50-60% by 2019, thanks to efforts to raise public awareness of Celiac disease.[9]
- ✓ Gluten-free sales are expected to reach $2.8 billion by the end of 2010 thanks to new vendors manufacturing better tasting and more affordable products.[10]

Gluten intolerance is not going away. It has become a largely ignored national problem for way too long. So many people have no idea that what they eat can harm their bodies in ways that extend well beyond just making you fat, which is all anyone seems to think about when they go grocery shopping. By understanding what Celiac disease is, you are taking the first step towards promoting a national change of attitude about what it really means to eat right. If you want to learn more about what it means to be gluten intolerant, or educate yourself on the digestive "ins and outs" of gastrointestinal functions, I highly recommend visiting the Celiac.com website for a number of remarkable explanations about what goes on inside of us when we eat. And, as you will see with my own crash course in learning

---

[9] Datamonitor Group, 2009.

[10] Gluten-free sales reached more than $2.6 billion by the end of 2010 and are now expected to exceed more than $5 billion by 2015. Packaged Facts, 2011.

to deal with Celiac disease, you can become more healthy and fit than you ever could have possibly imagined!

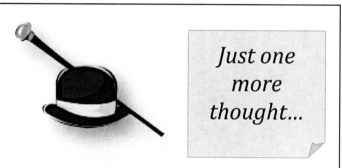

*Just one more thought...*

Do you think that Charlie Chaplin could have been a celiac? He usually walked in a penguin-like fashion and clenched his butt cheeks tightly to keep an accident from happening. Eureka!

I remember that bit when he used two dinner rolls on the tip of two forks to fashion a burlesque dance doing the Can-Can. At the conclusion of all of these scenes, maybe he ate the dinner rolls and ended up doing the "silent film shuffle" to the water closet? I don't remember reading any of the subtitles where he talked about needing a new pair of underwear from the wardrobe department, but you never know...

# Chapter Five

## There Will Be Blood

It took me months and months to discover that it was wheat doing all that damage to my insides. I visited my doctor several times to find out what was wrong with me. We didn't have much luck with discovering my ailment. Well, right before I left for Germany, my doctor conducted a full-fledged blood test to determine if I had any food allergies. All of the results came back negative. Unfortunately, he told me that I needed to think of an item or beverage that I eat each and every day and take that out of my diet for two weeks at a time.

Egads! The only foods I consumed daily that I could think of were anti-oxidants. Eliminating this from diet would not be easy by any means. I lived off of anti-oxidants. I also talked about their dietary benefits on TV when I was the Director of Marketing for Cedarlane Natural Foods. All of my favorite foods flashed before my eyes, and it pained me to think of how I would live without even one of them for fourteen days!

I loved them so much. Greek yogurt, eggs, blueberries, almonds, cranberries, coffee, dark chocolate, red wine, micro-brews, granola, oatmeal, fish, nuts, meats, tea, milk, organic burritos, pretzels, and cheese…just whittling down this list was going to take me half a year! I didn't seem to have a choice. I started with the main culprits that caused so many customers to call into the manufacturer where I worked.

I went for two weeks without fish, but that didn't stop it. Next, I moved onto all of my favorite dairy products, such as half & half, cottage cheese, yogurt, milk, and cheese, but that didn't do the trick either. Then I remembered a young woman who I worked with at Bozell Worldwide Advertising Agency in Chicago who was allergic to nuts. One day while at work, her father visited her after a Cubs afternoon game. He was a die-hard fan, which meant that his afternoon consisted of several Old

Style beers and a Rambo-like bag of peanuts. His visit was very much welcomed by all of us, but when he went to give his daughter a goodbye kiss, her nut allergy was so severe that his embrace landed her in the emergency room. That memory made me think: was I allergic to nuts?

I went through my kitchen, desk drawers, backpack, and every one of my snack hiding places. Bags and bags of nuts and peanut butter went into the garbage can. Once again, the euphoria set in as I specifically remember all of the horror stories of people calling our manufacturing plant and insisting that we divulge if there were even the slightest bit of nut ingredients in our formulas. They simply wanted to ensure that we weren't going to fast track them to the emergency room. Even though I gave up every nut imaginable over the next two weeks, I kept going into the bathroom almost two dozen times per day. Still…no answer.

After nearly six months of trial and error, I hadn't made the discovery of what was making me so ill, fatigued, and not able to put on lean muscle. I had an international trip planned for my upcoming birthday and wanted desperately to figure out what was wrong with me before my departure. My trip included flying to Munich, Germany, and I was hoping to "Om-Pah-Pah" at Oktoberfest without having to exit my lederhosen like Houdini from a straightjacket two dozen times per day. It was tough enough just to get a zipper down on a pair of dress pants, but try undoing the buckles, antler-boned buttons, and cross leather straps of a traditional Bavarian garb! This was going to be a rough vacation for sure.

Once again, I called the doctor for yet another office visit, this time the day of my trans-Atlantic flight. The doctor was speechless after looking at my six months of food elimination journal. Finally, his face turned sullen and he uttered the following words: "Unfortunately, I think I know what the problem is and what you need to do next. I need to get something out of my office in the other room and I will be right back." I didn't have a good feeling hearing those words come out of his mouth. I was supposed to be excited about leaving for the country where my great grandparents were born and buried—not considering my own burial proceedings!

After what seemed like an eternity, he came back into the room with a small business card and said:

> **"I am referring you to a gastroenterologist who specializes in internal diseases from the mouth to the anus."**

Suddenly, every awful scenario immediately crossed my mind: cancer, organ failure, internal parasite, bleeding, tumors, etc. They all seemed to be very real possibilities as to what was wrong with me. I started to sweat profusely. Was I going to die from this…whatever this was?

Being the optimist that I am, I told my doctor that I would make an appointment with the specialist once I returned from Germany. I went home, packed, grabbed my passport, and headed to the airport.

Most people get on an airplane worrying about getting a window seat or aisle seat. During the pre-celiac diagnosis days, I was the rare one who would specifically ask for a seat closest to the restroom. Yet, having a seat in close proximity to the toilet did nothing to ease my apprehension. Thankfully, I had made this transatlantic trip numerous times, thanks to my mother being a former TWA employee, and this seemed to ease my fear. I actually fell asleep as the airplane reached a cruising speed of 32,000 feet. In a matter of hours, I would be through customs at the airport and on my way to the Marienplatz (the square in the heart of Munich). Just the thought of being in Bavaria put me in a deep sleep on the plane. All that flour-and gluten-filled Bavarian food in front of me on a blue and white checked table in a *biergarten*...it can make any person's mouth water just thinking about it!

Little did I know, I was about to have a harsh revelation that gluten was the cause of my lifelong illness.

Defeat Wheat

# Chapter Six

## "Dude, What Happens to You When You Eat Gluten?"

I purposely wrote the first few chapters of this book with self-defecating…er… I mean self-*deprecating* humor. It's easy to look back and make fun of it now, but it wasn't funny at all trying to hide this embarrassing problem from everyone in my life. And most celiacs do just that. It's embarrassing that you have to take different routes in your office to the restroom each day so that people don't wonder why you are constantly in the restroom. Gluten turns us celiacs into diarrhea demons. Following the first sign that I'm about to explode, I literally feel like I am Superman crumpled in the fetal position and someone has put a bowling ball-sized rock of kryptonite around my neck. As the gluten makes its way out of the human body, it sucks out all of my energy. I'll crawl into bed and literally fall asleep in less than 15 seconds. I will then sleep for three hours straight without even waking, and this is after a full night's worth of sleep!

When I do get up, I feel like my head is one of those balloons in the Macy's Thanksgiving Day parade as it floats to and from the restroom. I have a sinus headache for the remainder of the day as well. Consequently, I've clocked quite a few sick days in the past two years thanks to gluten intolerance.

However, being gluten-free is not a choice, but a mandatory diet and lifestyle. Sure, I eat new things every month that will send me through the aforementioned fire drill, but I must continue to refine my diet to make sure it's wheat and gluten-free.

Once I was officially diagnosed, I went through two long months of defeating wheat. It was not easy and it certainly was a shock to my system. What got me through each day was the thought that this couldn't make things any worse for me. I would just have to keep looking for answers if this turned out to be another diagnostic cul-desac. *No big deal*, I said to myself. *I'm used to this crap* (pardon the pun)*!*

> Then, around the 60-day mark, something happened. Something amazing and completely unexpected. I started to see and feel incredible transformations with my body.

## Muscle Tone

- My abs were more defined than ever before.
- The weight that I was able to lift in the gym was increasing at a high rate.
- My shoulders and arms improved their muscle definition.

## Energy

- I could run further, faster, and longer.
- My energy levels went through the roof, and it became evident in my passion for the work that I did for my clients.

## Appearance

- I had to pull my belt a little bit tighter as my pants became more loose fitting.
- My skin became healthier looking and more vibrant.
- My body fat was tested at my local gym, and it was one of the lowest that they had ever seen.
- Random people were approaching me in the gym and asking me what I changed in my diet and work-out routine.

## Mind

- My mental alertness throughout the day and into the evening remained consistently high.
- My daily mood seemed to stay stable throughout the day with no more peaks and valleys.

My life improved in more ways than I ever could have thought possible. For the first time ever, I could be described as a "healthy" individual! Yet, it wasn't a miracle, and it didn't require me to have surgery, be on medication permanently, or learn a crazy dietary meal system attached to a merciless exercise regimen. All I did was give up gluten, and from this I became a new person and wouldn't even recognize my old self if he were standing right next to me.

Giving up gluten is not a bad thing at all. In fact, I still wonder why the word "disease" is attached to the definition of "Celiac." All the improvements in my health and body after giving up gluten for just sixty days made my diagnosis a cause for celebration.

This change also brings me back to an important lesson I learned earlier in life. Back in my advertising career, I was very fortunate to have worked on the first TV commercials for Sam's Club in Bentonville, Arkansas. We've all heard stories about Sam Walton and how his philosophy is instilled in their business practices. When you enter the corporate offices of Wal-Mart or SAM'S club, the halls are peppered with inspiring quotes from Mr. Walton. One quote in particular comes to mind:

> **There is no such thing as a problem; it's actually an opportunity.**

Opportunity. That man sure knew how to look at life differently than the rest of us. While one person sees a situation negatively, another sees it in a positive way. It's been a few years since being diagnosed as a celiac, and I believe that I was given an opportunity through my diagnosis to not only live a healthier lifestyle, but also show others how to do the same. Regardless if you're a celiac or not, you'll reap the rewards that numerous people have found when they eliminate wheat and gluten from their diets. And, if you continue to follow my plan, perhaps one day someone will approach you and ask, "What happens to you when you *don't* eat wheat?"

Your reply will be, "Why don't you grab a seat? This is going to be a *very* long conversation."

# Chapter Seven

## And, the Academy Award Goes To…

I have received numerous emails and letters from people who have had the same trials and tribulations as I did. What's interesting is that there is so much congruency with their life stories and my experiences as a celiac. Whenever I have written back to these people, there is always one resounding theme: we all should have received an academy award for acting normal when we actually felt like absolute sloths. One of these days, I would love to have our own acting awards program televised live on national TV. Perhaps we could call it the "Gluten Globes." If you have been in any of these situations as a celiac, you will know exactly what I am talking about:

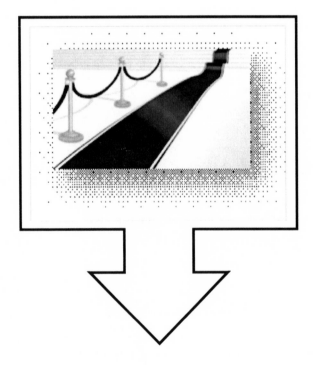

Ø Best Leading Actor/Actress in a business meeting: You feel like your head is one of those balloons in the Macy Thanksgiving Day parade, yet you hit the power point presentation on the "head."

Ø Best Visual Effects: How wonderful the "Restrooms →" sign looks when you are in a public place and moments away from having a celiac moment.

Ø Best Director: The method that you use to "cut" a personal visit or phone call short in order to make a bee line for the restroom.

Ø Best Costume Design: You've found a creative way to "hide the evidence" with a scarf, jacket, or long coat.

Ø Best Supporting Actor/Actress: You feel like Superman with a rock of kryptonite around your neck in the morning, but you meet your workout partner at the gym anyways despite the pain.

Ø Best Original Score: The sound of your stomach, upper intestines, and lower intestines as they play a symphony just before the dam opens.

Ø Best Animated Feature: Your cartoon mad dash to the aircraft bathroom the second that the "buckle your seatbelt" light goes off.

Let's face it: celiacs are a nation of actors and actresses. Whether we are in front of a classroom, across the table from a customer, to the left of a family member at a dinner, behind a microphone, connected to a telephone, or crossing a finish line, we still have this desire to hide our energy levels and feelings.

I'm sure that all of you have come across a hypochondriac in life. Well, hypochondriacs will tell you that they are ill 365 days a year, but celiacs will not feel well and play it off for years. We will chug along in our business meetings and in our personal lives as if we were well and that our energy levels were through the roof. This is just an act though. We accept that we must feel miserable, and some of us even accepted it knowing that there had to be some type of culprit responsible.

It was difficult for me to understand my diagnosis at first. I was the only person that I knew who had Celiac disease. I still kept up the "Best Actor" award for a long time and continued to hide the truth from everyone. You almost feel needy or embarrassed to talk about your ailment to business associates, friends, or strangers.

Likewise, there were many times that I would go to a business dinner at a restaurant and just pick and choose in the menu without asking for gluten-free alternatives. The worst was getting invited to a neighbor's house or out with a business acquaintance for dinner and struggle with telling them that I couldn't eat anything with gluten in it. Would that make me seem needy? Wouldn't I be seen as a painful guest who is mandating what should be served to me? And, how weak do I appear in front of a bunch of customers when I ask about specific ingredients in every appetizer, soup, entrée, side, and dessert? For a guy in sales, being a celiac was still embarrassing, despite my achievements in the gym and the board room.

So what did I do? I continued competing for a best actor award!

Business dinners were the worst. I would order entrees with sauces not knowing that they contained gluten. I dined on group appetizers chosen by everyone else at the table so as to look normal. I had dessert for special occasions that appeared to be nearly 100% wheat free, only to find myself in bed and in a gluten coma the next day.

You would think that I would have had the courage to simply ask the host or waiter about the contents of every item that appealed to me, but nobody wants to be an outcast. I wanted to look and act like everyone else and be a great restaurant guest and patron. I'm also not a nitpicky person about food. Growing up with parents that owned a restaurant will do that to you. I was supposed to *love* food. Yet, here I was being forced to play the role of an outcast with restrictive dietary needs! So, it got me thinking, *Am I the only one who feels this way?*

I did some research and found a statistic that put things into perspective for me: 1 in 133 Americans are afflicted with Celiac disease, according to the *Archives of Internal Medicine*, February 2003. This means I'm not alone!

To put it another way: an average Boeing 737 airplane holds about 150 people, and a typical big-city restaurant or gym on a busy night also holds about 150 people. Most floors in a large office have about 150 people working on them, too. This means there are people everywhere that are gluten intolerant. Consequently, I finally came to the realization that the benefits of me feeling on top of the world outweighed the perspective of me being an outsider.

If 1 in 133 people have Celiac disease, then how much of an outsider was I really? And so what if I seemed like this overly needy individual on that plane, gym, office floor, or restaurant? I had a proven formula for feeling good, and my overall stamina and strength was through the roof! I was done pretending like I didn't feel well. I decided to swear off gluten based items once and for all. I took a stand and to this day, I'm still standing.

# Chapter Eight

## Who Are the Celiacs In Your Neighborhood?
## (You Are Not Alone.)

I know plenty of foodies and people that love eating above all else, so I started asking the local food magazine writers and restaurant owners where I live if they were seeing a trend in the number of people requesting gluten-free foods. I also asked them if they personally knew of anyone with Celiac disease. I was suddenly introduced to people in my neighborhood who have Celiac disease and, surprisingly, they all live within a five mile radius of me!

For example, meet Julie, who lives only 100 yards from my house. Shortly after having children in her late 30's, she experienced a number of bodily problems. She was feeling more tired than ever, but chalked this up to time well-spent with her kids. However, the constant fatigue was also coupled with an enormous amount of gas throughout the day and accentuated by dizzy spells. Julie found herself giving up reading books, too. One paragraph would put her to sleep almost immediately. This perpetual cycle of lethargy eventually became unbearable.

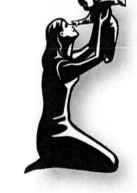

Around this time, her two sisters had been diagnosed with Celiac disease. Julie had to acquaint herself with the causes of Celiac disease and how to live with it, as she really had no idea what it meant to be a celiac. Shortly thereafter, her nieces were diagnosed with the same condition. *Could a gluten issue run in the family?* Julie wondered.

It was hard for Julie to stay both positive and healthy. Each morning, she would look down at the drain in her shower and notice entire clumps of hair. Not just a few hairs here and there, but enough to clog the drains every week! It was at this point Julie decided to schedule an appointment with her doctor.

Sure enough, the test for Celiac disease came back positive. The smallest instance of gluten in her lower intestines had wiped out her villi and her ability to absorb necessary vitamins and minerals. Her doctor went on to explain that her hair loss was due to malnutrition and that she needed to change her eating habits right away. Hence, Julie immediately adopted a gluten-free lifestyle and positive results started to appear within two weeks. New villi in her lower intestines were created, allowing her to absorb nutrients and replenish her body with essential vitamins and minerals needed for healthy living. She felt that her energy level basically doubled within the first month. Her overall mood improved drastically, and she didn't have late night fatigue anymore. Things were looking up—*way up*!

Julie's most significant change was the inclusion of weekly workouts at Red Rocks Amphitheater. For those of you unfamiliar with Red Rocks, it is an outdoor concert venue just west of Denver that is nestled in the foothills of the Rocky Mountains. The rocks around the stage have formed the perfect acoustical setting for numerous rock concerts, orchestras, and bands. When a concert is not in session, Julie works out on the stairs in the audience seating area. These stairs are about 6,000 feet above sea level. When you add up all of the stairs from the parking lot up to the last row, there are 388 in all. That's quite a Stairmaster! Julie works out for three and half hours there each week.

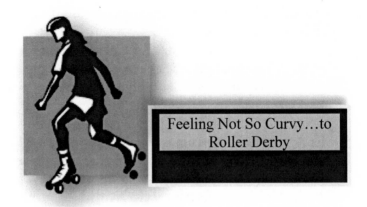

Feeling Not So Curvy…to
Roller Derby

Gabby is another neighbor of mine. She lives near the Rocky Mountains, just a few blocks south of Julie's home. At the age of 26, Gabby said "I do". It was supposed to be a great moment for her; however, her first year of marriage brought out the worst in both her husband and her bowels. She constantly fought and argued with her husband. She also started getting excruciating stomach pains after eating almost anything. These pains were sometimes accompanied by vomiting and utter fatigue. She wondered, *What the heck is going on?*

Well, Gabby knew it took two to tango, and with her husband it was just a matter of not seeing eye-to-eye on what they wanted in life. But, what was the reason for the newfound proverbial thorn in her side? Gabby initially thought she was eating food that was either spoiled or didn't agree with her stomach, so she didn't change her diet at all and dealt with the symptoms hoping that they would eventually go away. Only they didn't go away. They got worse.

Christmas Day of 2007 was spent in the Emergency Room with pains so unbearable she thought someone had thrown a ten pound shot put made of fruitcake right into her abdomen. The ER staff performed every test imaginable, including an ultrasound. All of the tests confirmed that she was a "healthy" woman. I guess that would be the kind of gift Gabby would want on Christmas, but the pain still wasn't going away.

The other "gifts" that she received around the holidays were compliments from family and friends about her visible weight loss. Except Gabby wasn't on a diet. She accepted the kind remarks anyways and continued to watch her dress size shrink rapidly. She didn't see this as a good thing, though. It was an alarming fifty pound weight loss in the space of a few months!

By autumn of 2008, Gabby was also spending an enormous amount of time going to the bathroom. It was after one of these relief visits that Gabby took a hot shower to relax and release some residual tension. After the shower, she noticed something terrible had happened. Her hair had fallen out in clumps and was clogging the drain. This was the breaking point. Gabby immediately sought help.

Her search led to a gastroenterologist, who performed a rudimentary blood test that came back positive for Celiac disease. Not being fully aware of what it meant, Gabby knew that the word "disease" attached to it couldn't be good news. She took comfort, though, knowing that the specialist was very up to date on the recent trend of celiac cases. In fact, the specialist had told her that having Celiac disease was manageable! The doctor explained that being a celiac meant following a gluten-free diet. When Gabby asked what this involved, he proceeded to tell her all the things she could and couldn't eat. It was scary to think about drastically changing her diet, but if this meant not suffering anymore tear-soaked bowel spasms and embarrassing ER visits, she had to try.

Within weeks of changing her dietary habits, her energy levels improved and her hair had stopped falling out. Her marriage was still on the rocks, but Gabby's life became tolerable once again.

It wasn't until a few months after her diagnosis that the stomach pains resurfaced. She couldn't believe what was happening, so she went back to the specialist again with a copy of her gluten-free diet to prove her strict adherence to a gluten-free diet. The doctor told her it would take time for the villi to grow back in the lower intestines and that perhaps that was the culprit. Gabby had also described a different type of pain she was feeling on top of the familiar gut tremors. Her doctor decided to take an MRI to look for additional issues.

Unfortunately, the MRI found a few cysts on her ovaries. The doctor had suspected these were in her body for quite some time. According to him, the ovarian cysts "ebb and flow" in size depending upon a woman's menstrual cycle. He assumed that the cysts were probably there prior to the celiac diagnosis but had gone undetected because they were much smaller at the time.

As if this wasn't enough, Gabby reflected on the fact that she had just started a very demanding new job as a Colorado water resource manager. Her body had been through dietary torture, and her marriage was a nightmare as well. Now cysts? Enough was enough. Gabby got rid of three of the most malignant things in her life: her husband, those damn cysts, and gluten.

She subsequently followed a very strict diet and read every celiac cook book she could get her hands on. She also opted to not be put on any prescription drugs. Instead, she used food as her medicine. Two months later, her energy levels were through the roof and she was as mentally and physically fit as a teenager!

This newfound energy also provided just the push she needed to join the Denver Roller Dolls derby league. Gabby gave it all she had, and it wasn't long before she would be drafted to play for the Bad Apples. Her achievements with the Bad Apples earned her a coveted spot playing for Colorado's top-ranked competitive Roller Derby All-star team known as the Mile High Club.

Her athletic skill also earned her the coveted MVP award during the 2009 national championship for the Denver Roller Dolls. As if this wasn't enough, she battled her way up the ranks until reaching the Mile High Club's coveted status of "Captain." Gabby still plays to this day.

If you haven't seen a roller derby bout, it is one of the world's most physically challenging sports. With at least five hours of practices a week under their belts, these derby girls are fierce in their determination to win matches. So, the next time you are in the Mile High City, come see the Denver Roller Dolls in full tilt boogie. If I could pick somebody to defend the nation from gluten, a roller derby girl is my first choice.

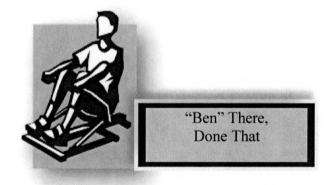

"Ben" There, Done That

I first met Ben at our local gym a few years ago. We are both such early risers that there were mornings when it would be just the two of us working out. Before I even knew his name or background, it was very easy to determine that he probably played football in college (due to his thickness), but, like most post-college football players, a number of factors had physically changed his body: new jobs, marriage, meeting schedules, travel, change in metabolism, and little understanding of diet. With that said, Ben was probably several pounds heavier than what he would like to be. I'm sure that "back in the day" he was ripped!

When we started talking to each other on a first name basis at the gym, I had just been diagnosed with Celiac disease. Ben had watched my subsequent progress for six months with wheat and gluten eliminated from my diet. After the first three months, he finally cornered me and said, "What gives with you? I do aerobic training every other day in hopes of cutting fat, and I lift the other days to build muscles. Yet you are the one getting leaner and building more muscle every single week, and I know it because I'm the one spotting your bench presses and adding the weight plates onto the lift bars. Meanwhile, it's *my* belly that keeps growing!"

I told him that I had been diagnosed with Celiac disease. He gave me the usual perplexed look, the one where fifty percent of the look is one of sorrow based on the assumption that you have some sort of fatal illness. The other fifty percent is confusion about what Celiac disease is. Once I explained what gluten was and why it adversely affects millions of people, Brian initiated the following exchange of words:

"So no bread?" Ben asked me.

"Nope. Well, unless it's gluten-free bread," I replied.

"No pasta?" as he scratched his chin.

"No."

"What about beer?"

"Unfortunately no, unless it's a special gluten-free beer. And believe me, I didn't know that last Halloween and it was truly the most terrifying holiday that I have ever had," I said.

He paused, then said, "Well, that sucks."

My reply to this and anything that you don't have control over is, "It could be much worse."

Over the next several weeks, Ben told me that he discussed both my Celiac disease and post-diagnosis progress with his wife. She immediately thought about the fact that her husband was eating more than his fair share of wheat from dawn to dusk. Even though he wasn't showing signs of being gluten intolerant, she began to suspect his wheat and gluten intake as being the primary reason for his added fat and ever growing belly.

Ben's wife suggested that he talk to me about how he could possibly manage his weight by cutting out gluten. I discussed in detail with Ben how I was building my meals throughout the day and re-thinking all my food choices. I could tell by the look on his face that this was information overload. Being a seasoned ex-advertising agent, I told him that I would put together a power point presentation and email it to him over the next few days. He laughed at this suggestion but agreed to it anyways. (We advertising guys just *love* making power point presentations!)

I developed two of my dieting programs into visual diagrams, both of which can be found and further explained in Chapters 13-15. Ben was my first client to follow them. He printed off three separate copies for home, work, and the gym.

Cutting out gluten was not an easy task the first month, especially on Sundays when he watched football and was surrounded with beer and pizza. Ben didn't waiver, though. He stuck to eliminating all gluten from his diet until something happened that his wife noticed even before he did. He was shedding pounds every week. It wasn't too long before his wife complimented him daily on how finely sculpted his body looked, causing Ben's self-confidence to soar through the roof.

After giving up gluten, Ben had lost a total of 36 pounds. Was Ben a celiac? I sincerely doubt it. Did he reap the benefits of giving up wheat and gluten? I think if you ask his wife, the resounding answer would be yes!

## Take Down

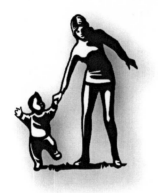

Once all of my neighbors found out that I was writing a book on living gluten-free, I started receiving numerous phone calls and emails from people who were interested in my transformation. That is how I met Trudy and her fifteen year-old son Tyler.

Being a working mother, Trudy has relied on daycare to help her through the busy weeks. While at the daycare, Tyler had little interest in anything athletic during playtime or recess. He chose to stay inside and focus on reading and writing. Sometime after this, Tyler began having asthma attacks. Some of these attacks were severe, but whenever they went to the hospital, his oxygen levels were always found to be between the normal range of 95-100%. Still, his condition was so debilitating that he had trouble even getting out of bed.

As if being a toddler wasn't hard enough, uncontrollable diarrhea started happening in and out of the class room. He had a particularly scary episode where, after coming home from eating pizza with some friends, he began stumbling and walking around the house in a zombie-like manner. This lasted for three days and then mysteriously disappeared. Sometime after this happened, Tyler had another episode shortly after eating again at one of his favorite restaurants. This time the symptoms were diarrhea, stomach cramps, lethargy, dizziness, nausea, conjunctivitis, bloodshot eyes, and vomiting. He actually slept for three days straight. Trudy took him to the ER for dehydration and the doctors said it was gastroenteritis and gave him an IV before sending him home.

Tyler seemed to continue visiting the ER every six months as a result of what the doctors called gastroenteritis. At age ten, he suddenly gained weight, started sleeping 14-15 hours a day, and his energy level became dangerously low. He still remained a good student, but his decreased level of movement caused him to develop a shuffling gait, making it difficult to walk or run like other kids. The counselor at school believed Tyler had A.D.D. When Trudy had him tested, the interviewing specialists said he was suffering from depression, not A.D.D.

Well, neither diagnosis made sense to Trudy. Tyler didn't act depressed or apathetic, he acted sick and lethargic. The specialists strongly advised Tyler to exercise no matter how difficult it was for him. Trudy followed the physician's orders and harassed her poor son to do mile-long walks around the lake near their home. He complained about his legs and feet continuously hurting from these physically demanding treks and eventually ended up being unable to attend school due to exhaustion. Every physical action also took extreme effort and he was becoming more frustrated each day. He continually asked his mother, "Why can't I play and run like other kids?" Trudy didn't have an answer. She didn't know what to tell her son for the next six years of his life.

Two weeks before Tyler turned sixteen year-old, Trudy discovered the truth about her son: he had Celiac disease. It was as if the proverbial light bulb turned on and illuminated what was really happening to her child. All of his bouts with illness could be celiac-related. She had also read that asthma is a symptom of a severe vitamin D deficiency, which is quite common in celiacs. Trudy had to be sure, so she prescribed Tyler a gluten-free diet and in just four days, he was feeling better. Three months into being gluten-free, his muscles and joints didn't hurt anymore. His asthma also disappeared, and his strength and ability to walk began returning to normal.

Upon seeing these signs of improvement with Tyler, Trudy reached out to me for suggestions on planning gluten-free meals. She wanted to know about strength training and building muscle mass as well. I went to work and came up with a plan for her, one that included jogging for long periods of time. Tyler didn't even flinch at my plan. He delved right into it and became consistently active for the first time ever in his life. He has told me that nothing hurts anymore and he actually enjoys performing physical activities, including lifting weights and working out at the gym. He doesn't sleep excessively either, and his attitude reflects a growing optimism intertwined with positivity.

Trudy feels that Celiac disease stole her son's childhood, but thanks to a gluten-free lifestyle, he has been given a chance to be reborn again.

# Chapter Nine

## Give Blood ~
## Your Benchmark Test

W hile working with Dr. Barry Sears, creator of the "Zone Diet," for more than a year at Cedarlane, I learned the deep importance of getting your blood tested at least once a year. I have attended several lectures where Dr. Sears explains the phenomena of "classic inflammation," where you feel actual pain and this prompts a visit to the doctor's office.[11] Along with this, there is the phenomena of "silent inflammation," which is below the perception of pain. Because you can't feel silent inflammation, it can continue to attack your internal organs without you even knowing it. Celiacs are a good example of people who suffer from this unfelt pain. The villi in a celiac's stomach are attacked and eventually wiped out, malnutrition sets in, and the celiac will have had no idea it ever happened until it's too late.

Do you see then why it's important to get a blood test? You may be a victim of silent inflammation! Getting a blood test will provide you with a snapshot of your overall health. I actually have my blood tested two times per year!

Let me restate this again, because it's SO IMPORTANT:

> The first step toward finding out if you have a gluten intolerance or Celiac disease is for you to have your blood taken and analyzed.

---

[11] Sears, Barry. *The Anti-Inflammation Zone: Reversing the Silent Epidemic That's Destroying Our Health*. Regan Books. 2005.

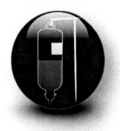

Whether you decide to eliminate wheat from your diet or dramatically reduce it, you and your doctor can use the blood test as a starting point. Do you think that your blood test will just show your cholesterol and blood sugar levels? Think again. It can tell you many things about your overall well being.

Don't fret if there are some irregularities in certain areas, though. Some of them can be normal. For instance, you may have a high blood sugar count from eating fresh fruit less than ten hours before the blood is drawn, as fresh fruits contain natural sugars. You may also come up with a false negative for Celiac disease but still have it!

So, go ahead and schedule an appointment with your doctor for that blood test. I know this sounds weird, but you're going to start looking forward to these blood tests every six months. Whenever I get my results, I feel like a school kid running home from the bus stop with an exceptional report card clenched in both hands and ready to show the world! My tests repeatedly demonstrate the positive value of eating gluten-free food. I feel like my outside appearance is congruent with how I look on the inside, too. In fact, blood reminds us all that our bodies are engines with food and beverage as its fuel. The more wholesome and balanced your diet is, the better your fat-fighting ability will increase.

# Chapter Ten

## The Basic Principles of Food Selection

A few years ago, I was the spokesperson and on-air talent for the inaugural line of Zone Diet frozen foods on the QVC shopping network. People would call in and ask questions about dieting, food, and eating right. One question in particular I was asked over and over again was, "How do I read the food labels so that I can shop in a healthier manner?" (See "Ex. 1" on page 85)

I'm sure that you have asked this question many times yourself. My answer is simple:

> **If you read each line on a food label and see very long words that you have no clue what they are, put the food item back on the shelf.**

These days, food manufacturers are loading packaged foods with artificial flavors, texture enhancers, and preservatives that would make any of us feel clueless. If you don't know why something is being added to food, let alone pronounce the ingredient's name, why would you put it into your body? It doesn't make sense to me, and I want to talk some sense into you. Here are some of the ingredients I'm talking about:

- ✓ **Acesulfame K:** Sugar substitute found in pudding, chewing gum, non-dairy creamers, instant coffee mixes, tea mixes, and gelatin desserts. May increase cancer in humans.
- ✓ **Aspartame:** A genetically modified, synthetic sugar substitute found as a sweetener in diet sodas, cereal, chewing gum, juices, peas, and yogurt. People report dizziness, headaches and even seizures eating food containing this ingredient. Scientists believe it can also alter behavior due to impaired brain function. Long term effects of this genetically modified organism on human health has not been studied or tested.
- ✓ **High Fructose Corn Syrup/HFCS:** High fructose consumption has been fingered as a causative factor in heart disease. It raises blood levels of cholesterol and triglycerides. It makes blood cells more prone to clotting, and it may also accelerate the aging process. Found primarily in soda and breads, cereals, and candy bars, to name a few.
- ✓ **Hydrogenated/Partially Hydrogenated Oils:** Hydrogenated oils contain high levels of trans fat, which is an otherwise normal fatty acid that has been radically changed by high heat. They are pure poison (just like arsenic)! Partially hydrogenated oils are just as bad, as they will slowly kill you over time. They help produce diseases like multiple sclerosis and allergies that lead to arthritis, and will also make you fat! Found in fast foods, snack foods, fried foods, and baked goods.

✓ **Monosodium Glutamate/MSG:** MSG is an excitotoxin, which causes nerve damage and allergic reactions. Found in hundreds of foods, such as salad dressings, canned prepared foods, seasonings, and bouillon cubes, often under another name, Sodium Glutamate.

✓ **Nitrate /Nitrite:** While nitrate itself is harmless, it is readily converted to nitrite. When nitrite combines with compounds called secondary amines, it forms nitrosamines. These are extremely powerful cancer-causing chemicals. The chemical reaction occurs most readily at the high temperatures of frying. Cured meats are a prime example. Nitrite has long been suspected as being a cause of stomach cancer as well.

✓ **Sodium Nitrite:** Makes meat look red rather than gray, and gives meat an overly long shelf life of months. Sodium Nitrite is clinically proven to cause leukemia, brain tumors, and other forms of cancer.

✓ **Potassium Sorbate:** A preservative used to inhibit molds and yeasts in many foods, such as soft drinks and fruit drinks, snacks, and baked goods.

✓ **Sodium Benzoate:** Same as Potassium Sorbate in its ability to lengthen food and beverage shelf lives.

As you start to eliminate wheat from your diet, you're also going to eliminate ingredients that have way too many letters and are way too difficult to pronounce. It's amazing how much gluten and these ingredients are linked to unhealthy food. Just remember:

> ## You Are What You Eat

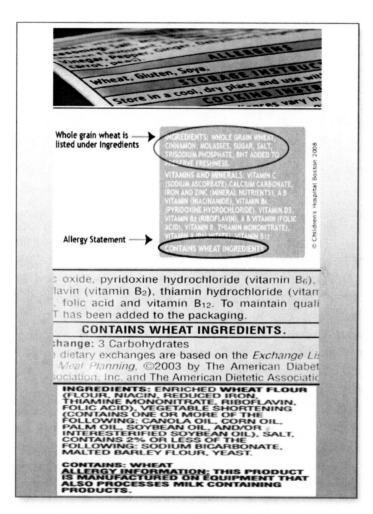

Ex. 1: How to Read Labels[12]

---

[12]http://www.fda.gov/Food/LabelingNutrition/FoodLabelingG
uidanceRegulatoryInformation/InformationforRestaurantsRetailEstablis
hments/ucm063367.htm

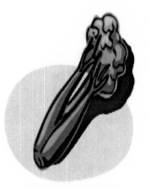

# The Celery Stalk Experiment

Twice a year, the all natural and organic food industry has two major food shows. The larger west coast show is called Expo West and the much smaller east coast show is called Expo East. I would highly recommend that you make a visit to either one of them for a better understanding about where the food industry is headed. Not only are the convention centers full of trade show booths with all natural and organic foods, they are full of presentations that clearly demonstrate the increasing benefits of eating "clean."

I'm certain to get a few calls and e-mails from food industry officials who can give you a laundry list of why chemicals help accentuate the growth of national crops and are actually good for you. Well, they can show me all of the empirical data in the world, but their supposed evidence only brings me back to a science experiment I did in Catholic grade school that supports the idea of "less is more" with food ingredients.

I was in fifth grade and learning about osmosis. All the students were told to bring a stalk of celery to school for the lesson. It looked like a bizarre scene from a movie, seeing everyone on the bus carrying huge stalks of celery wrapped with aluminum foil at the base. We arrived at school, and the teacher divided us into teams, giving each team a beaker filled with water. The teacher then asked us to put our celery stalks into the containers. When we were finished doing this, she walked around to every group and put a few drops of red food coloring into each container. Each group was given the final instruction to put their beakers on the shelf in the back of the room, where they would remain overnight.

The next day when we arrived in science class, portions of the celery stalks clearly had a pink tint! Our teacher explained the reason for this was osmosis and how water moves through membranes. I was amazed. At the conclusion of the experiment, she asked if we had any questions. I raised my hand.

"Does that mean that we're actually eating all of the fertilizers I've seen the farmers spray on their fields as we ride the bus to school?"

That day in class I not only learned about osmosis, but I learned what a "blank stare" was, too. It was the first time in my young life I had asked a question that left a teacher speechless. She ignored me and proceeded to ask the rest of the class if there were any other questions about the experiment. I took her response as a "yes."

I'm not going to debate whether or not those chemicals actually are ingested into your system, but the celery stalk experiment proves that we eventually become what we eat. You have a choice each and every day to make healthy food decisions. There are hundreds, if not thousands, of food and beverage items in your local store that are "all natural," "organic," or "preservative free." So read the ingredients on the packages and as a general rule, select those items with the least number of ingredients.

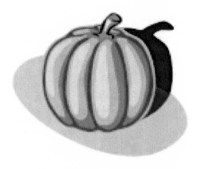

# The Port of Produce

When you walk into most grocery stores, the produce section is typically the first area you'll see. This is a very good place to start. I want you to think about the produce department as the "Port of Produce." I don't even need to tell you about the health benefits of eating multiple servings of fresh fruits and vegetables a day. All of us need to eat more produce, but we always seem to find some sort of an excuse not to buy or eat it.

I worked directly with the Produce for Better Health Foundation when I was at my second advertising agency. This is an exceptional non-profit organization that encourages consumers to pre-plan their produce purchases. Elizabeth Pivonka , the P.B.H. President and C.E.O. and one of the P.B.H.'s registered dieticians, states that:

> As a registered dietitian and mom, the best advice I can give is to choose nutrient-dense foods that offer higher vitamin, mineral and fiber content per calorie like healthy fruits and vegetables and 100 percent fruit or vegetable juice to get as much nutritional bang for your buck as possible. Eating more of these foods in place of other items with added sugar and high fat content is the best way to lose or maintain weight, feel more energized, and stay healthy.

Later in the book, I will list the exact types of produce that should be added to your weekly shopping list. You are going to embark on your wheat free journey at the "Port of Produce." Indeed, Elizabeth Pivonka goes on to point out:

> First, leaf through your supermarket's latest ad flyer. This will show you what's on sale. Fresh fruits and vegetables that are in season will be at their peak of flavor and they're least expensive, so if you see some of your family's favorites at a bargain be sure to incorporate them into your menu plan. But don't worry if their favorites aren't in season that week. Canned and frozen fruits and veggies are just as nutritious as fresh and you can load up the pantry with them when they go on sale. Then, figure out which recipes you would like to prepare in the coming week. You'll use the list of on-sale items and your recipes' ingredients to build your shopping list for the week. By planning out your meals for the week, you know you'll have everything you need on hand to make a healthy meal that your family will enjoy.

Have you found yet another reason or excuse for not adding fresh produce to your grocery list? If so, I recommended ditching that excuse and loading your shopping carts with produce. After all, today's produce is safer than ever. Not sure what to buy? Don't be surprised at how knowledgeable produce employees are. They know which items sell best, which ones recently arrived, those that have received rave reviews from fellow customers, or when a new crop is due to arrive soon. Many times they will even cut open an item for you to try.

There is something else that makes "The Port of Produce" a great place to start your journey:

## It's GLUTEN-FREE!

# Are You Single? (Digit, That Is.) If So, We Have a Place to "Meat"

Many people who hear the word "diet" think that they can't eat any more meats they love. This isn't always true. If you are a carnivore, I have very good news. You are going to have some type of lean animal protein in nearly every one of your main meals. Unprepared and un-marinated meats and seafood are inherently gluten-free, and not only are they gluten-free, they are packed with protein that you'll need to get both cut and lean. So whether you are a celiac, are looking at reducing or eliminating wheat from your diet, or just want to get more toned, eating the proper meats will help you stay healthy and fit all the time.

First, you will need to research those animal proteins that have single digit fat content per serving. Not sure what a serving actually entails? Put it this way: a serving of three ounces is approximately the size of a deck of cards.

## Remember the Government Guidelines:

> - **Lean – Less than 10 grams of total fat, less than 4.5 grams of saturated fat, and less than 95 grams of cholesterol per 3 ounce serving.**
> - **Extra Lean – Less than 5 grams of total fat, less than 2 grams of saturated fat, and less than 95 grams of cholesterol per 3 ounce. serving.**

While preparing your shopping list for the week, look through your weekly circulars for good deals and preferably these cuts of lean meats:

| Beef Cuts 3 oz. portion (visible fat trimmed) | Calories | Saturated Fat (g) | Total Fat (g) |
|---|---|---|---|
| Eye Round Roast | 144 | 1.4 | 4.0 |
| Sirloin Tip Side Steak | 143 | 1.6 | 4.1 |
| Top Round Roast | 157 | 1.6 | 4.6 |
| Bottom Round Roast | 139 | 1.7 | 4.9 |
| Top Sirloin Steak | 156 | 1.9 | 4.9 |
| 95% Lean Ground Beef | 139 | 2.4 | 5.1 |

| Pork Cuts 3 oz. portion (visible fat trimmed) | Calories | Saturated Fat (g) | Total Fat (g) |
|---|---|---|---|
| Tenderloin | 120 | 1.0 | 3.0 |
| Boneless Top Loin Chops | 173 | 1.8 | 5.2 |
| Boneless Top Loin Roast | 147 | 1.6 | 5.3 |
| Center Loin Chops | 153 | 1.8 | 6.2 |
| Poultry Cuts 3 oz. portion (visible fat trimmed) | Calories | Saturated Fat (g) | Total Fat (g) |
| Skinless Chicken Breast | 140 | 0.9 | 3.1 |
| Ground Turkey Breast | 110 | 0.5 | 1.0 |

# For The Leanest Cuts of Meat…

During my advertising days in Chicago, I worked with clients to advertise beef entrees that were sold in their stores or restaurants. From the consumer focus groups that we conducted for Kroger grocery stores or the annual holiday catalog that we printed for SAM'S Club, we knew what would encourage the inclusion of meat into anyone's daily diet: a mouth-watering visual of a steak or roast with an ample amount of marbling. This certainly wasn't a crap shoot or a guess that consumers wanted this. We spent a great deal of time, resources, and money to get inside the brain of the typical American. It worked every time in boosting sales. Every single time.

Listen, you can forget everything that you may have learned about advertising from *Bewitched*, *Melrose Place*, or *Mad Men*. While the characters in the aforementioned shows are jumping into a three-martini lunch or into bed with a co-worker, the smartest advertising minds are jumping into stacks of proprietary consumer trends and information. To this day, the most successful agencies typically have a research director that holds the blueprint for consumer hot buttons. These were the people that would determine a designated set of M.S.P.'s (Main Selling Propositions) that would substantiate the Pavlov theory with consumers: marbling in meat makes consumers' mouths water and cash registers ring! Our research director actually interviewed tens of dozens of consumers and all of them equated flavor and quality with the marbling in a typical steak.

If you don't believe me, look at your favorite food magazines. Spot any raw prime rib that has so much marbling it looks like the highway roadmap for all of New England? What about ads for white table cloth restaurants where the servers parade around with silver platters holding all the succulent, sculptured raw meats imaginable? If you eat at a place like this, the wait staff will purposely point out all of the marbling and how it adds to the taste. Every patron in the room will invariably reply with "oohs" and "ahhs" as if they just saw an aerial fireworks display.

Marbling in an advertisement does work. It makes people's mouths water when they visualize the strains of fat in print or on TV. It also helps the waiter at that white table cloth restaurant sell you on the porter house cut. Heck, did I mention my parents' steak house? They keep a fully aged rib eye roast in their front lobby meat case and a fully cooked prime rib in the kitchen ready to slice. The prime rib sells by the ounce and it's one of the restaurant's most demanded cuts of meat.

The question still remains though: why do we like the marbling? Because, once the meat is cooked, the marbling is what makes the steak juicy and tasty. It's also why we Americans love butter and olive oil so much. The fat shepherds all of these different flavors to the tongue's sensory areas. Fat is what makes us say "yum" at the dining room table and it starts a party in our brain. What else does fat do?

Many healthcare experts will tell you that the visible fat on those steaks is what makes you fat. But, you can dramatically reduce the fat content with two simple tools: a knife and fork.

Make sure that you trim all visible fat from any cut of beef, chicken, or pork prior to preparation.[13] Additionally, opt for cuts that were mentioned in both of the previous beef and pork chart and you can be certain they are the leanest. If you want to get "the skinny" on what cuts to purchase, make copies of both charts that are in this chapter and use a paring knife to cut the fat from all your meat selections.

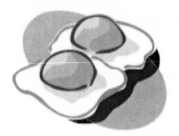

# The Incredible Edible Egg

What is a great source of protein that also allows you to start the day feeling guilt-free about food? EGGS, BABY! My sincere apologies if you have an egg allergy, but eggs are the bomb! You should try and eat them every single day if your schedule permits. Why am I so hot about eggs? Just look at the facts from the American Egg Board:[14]

---

[13] "A guide to choosing lean meats and poultry", *Nutrition & Weight Control*, August 20, 2008.
[14] www.aeb.org

- Each egg contains roughly 70 calories.
- Egg protein is the standard by which other protein sources are measured. A large egg contains over 6 grams of protein!
- Only one-third (1.5) grams is saturated fat and 2 grams are mono-unsaturated fat.
- The American Heart Association has amended its guidelines on eggs! There is no longer a specific recommendation on the number of egg yolks a person may consume in a week.
- A large egg has 4.5 grams of fat, only 7% of the daily value. Remember my reference to "Are you single?" Keep those fat grams in the single digit range.
- Eggs are rich in nutrients.

All of these benefits in one little egg shell. No wonder why more and more people choose eggs as a healthy addition to their diets.[15] And those usage numbers keep rising, according to the American Egg Board:

- Item penetration is very high, 93%, which means that eggs can be found in almost every household.
- Recent sales data is showing a positive rejuvenation of the egg category.
- Here's some great news! Consumer research conducted by Miller-Zell, a retail services and

---

[15] For further information, refer to, "Eggs are winners for grocery stores", Foodlink, Rod Smith 7/10/2010.

marketing strategy firm, revealed that the overwhelming majority (85%) of shoppers view eggs as very or somewhat healthy.

✓ Consumers like the versatility of eggs and the variety of dishes they can be used in. And, they are looking for information on delicious, nutritious meals which feature eggs as a major ingredient.

I am sure there is this little whisper in your ear saying, "Didn't I hear something about eggs being contaminated and that they contain some sort of bad bacteria?" I would highly recommend not letting any type of isolated egg incident decrease your confidence in the American agricultural system. In fact, there is a governing board called the United Egg Producers[16] that are dedicated to assuring that Americans can continue to buy eggs that are produced in a safe and environmentally sound method. U.E.P. certified guidelines pertain to both cage and cage-free housing systems, and this board is everything it's clucked up to be!

So don't forget to add eggs to your gluten-free diet.

---

[16] www.unitedegg.org

# Chapter Eleven

## Frozen Food Fanatic

I n the retail world, the "golden horseshoe" is the outside perimeter of every store where produce is mostly kept. This "Port of Produce" is jam-packed with fresh, gluten-free items. Once you finish buying all the produce you can handle, get your parka on because next we are heading into the frozen food section!

Today's frozen food section is unlike anything it was in the last century. You are not going to be eating from an aluminum foil punched-out tray that we older Gen-X'ers remember from the 70's and 80's. Thinking of the "olden days" of TV dinners reminds me of a commercial that I produced for Kroger called "Freezer Lady."

Long story short, the actress in the spot was preparing for the big Kroger frozen food sale. In order to get ready for the sale, she was going to make space by defrosting the layers of ice and frost that were in her freezer compartment above the refrigerator. As she started removing ice chunks frozen since the Nixon administration, she found her long lost vacuum cleaner attachment behind the ice maker. I know for a fact that Kroger customers related to it, based upon the copious fan mail that Kroger received.

There was one parallel to frozen foods from the days when I was in school and the vacuum cleaner attachment that the "Freezer Lady" found: they both sucked! At least, I thought so. Then again, my family has been in the restaurant business for over a quarter of a century, my brother is a trained chef, and my mother is the world's best cook. We didn't take entire meals out of the freezer on a nightly basis. We made everything from scratch. Whenever I did pull something from the freezer as a kid, the result was simply awful.

Still, there had to be a rhyme or reason for frozen foods' existence. How did it first come about? Why was it so awful last century? Why is it absolutely amazing today? And finally, what has made the nation's leading retailers commit more square footage toward freezer space today than ever before?

In order to answer the first question posed above, we need to get into Mr. Peabody's "way-back" time machine and head back to the Ice Ages. (Okay, not quite that far back, but I couldn't resist the pun.)

Believe it or not, some historians have actually found evidence that the ancient Chinese used ice cellars to preserve food through the cold winter months and beyond. The Romans stored food in compressed snow using insulated cellars as well. These early practices were a proven method of extending the life of food from earlier harvest seasons. As a result, the Chinese and Romans always had a reliable source of food that could be brought out of "hibernation" at a moment's notice. They were probably a lot like those of us who lead busy lives.

After all, who really wakes up each morning and knows exactly what they are going to have for lunch or dinner later that day? That's why we have these elaborate storage units in our garages and in our kitchens like the Chinese and the Romans did centuries ago.

The actual person given credit for the invention of modern frozen foods is American fur trader Clarence Birdseye.[17] In 1917, while he was fur-trading in Labrador, Canada, he noticed that the local residents would preserve fresh meat and fish by rapidly letting it freeze in Arctic temperatures. With the perfect combination of ice, wind, and low temperature, anything left exposed would freeze almost instantaneously. Mr. Birdseye also learned that this method of quick freezing kept ice crystals from forming on

---

[17] "Clarence Birdseye." Encyclopedia of World Biography. Vol. 19. 2nd ed. Detroit: Gale, 2004. 25-27. Gale Virtual Reference Library. Gale. Brigham Young University - Utah. Nov. 3 2009.

the ingredients that he was hoping to preserve in sub-zero temperatures.

Clarence perfected the first process for freezing the food. He did this with a simple electric fan, a few buckets of brine, and some large bricks of ice. A few years after this, frozen foods were sold to the public in 1929, and food experts hailed this innovation as a wonderful method of keeping a harvest fresh for prolonged periods of time in a stable environment. Little did Mr. Birdseye know that there were a variety of other benefits associated with freezing. According to the Frozen Food Foundation, there are four crucial benefits to choosing frozen foods:

## Frozen Foods are Nutritious

Did you know that frozen fruits and vegetables are processed within hours of harvest, thereby essentially "locking in" their vitamins and minerals? Raw products can spend several days or even weeks in transit or in storage prior to consumption, all the while losing key nutrients. In fact, researchers at the University of California Center for Excellence in Fruit and Vegetable Quality concluded that frozen fruits and vegetables are equally nutritious as their fresh and canned counterparts—and perhaps more so for some nutrients.[18]

The frozen food industry has also made great strides in improving the nutritional value of prepared foods. The recipes for many products now contain less fat, sugar, and sodium. Others make use of added fiber, contain zero trans-fat, and feature reduced portion sizes for sensible eating. All-natural frozen fruit smoothies are just a few of the

---

[18] "Maximizing the nutritional value of fruits and vegetables", Diane M. Barrett PhD, Director of the Center for excellence in fruit and vegetable quality, University of California Davis.

many examples of frozen food products that play an integral part in a healthy and well-balanced diet.

## Frozen Foods are a Real Value

Consumers find comfort in knowing they can prepare top-quality, restaurant-inspired meals at home at a fraction of the cost of eating out. But, value isn't just about dollars and cents; it's about delivering on consumers' expectations of quality and taste at a price that is affordable. Consumers are more often turning to the frozen food aisle to find great value. In fact, 2009 Perishables Group data suggests that among grocery shoppers who are looking to economize without sacrificing quality, 30% are buying more frozen foods than in previous years. Frozen products are also often lower in cost per serving and have a much greater shelf-life than refrigerated foods by their very nature. And, frozen fruits and vegetables can be more easily portioned and stored for use at a later time, which reduces spoilage and food waste. Single-serving pouches, re-sealable packs, and "servings for two" make it even easier for consumers to find a great value to suit their needs.

## Frozen Foods are Convenient

A 2008 Zogby International survey found that 87% of consumers purchase frozen foods because they are convenient and easy to prepare. And, it's no coincidence that some of the hottest products in the frozen food aisle are portable, ready-to-eat, and offer no-mess preparation and easy clean-up. All this built-in convenience means time-pressed moms and dads can quickly prepare wholesome and tasty meals that allow for more quality time spent around the table. Additionally, frozen fruits and vegetables come peeled, pre-cut, and ready to cook or eat. No washing or cutting is required, which saves time and reduces waste.

It's easy to toss your favorite frozen vegetables in with chicken and rice, or to pack a frozen fruit cup with a brown bag lunch.

## Freezing is a Natural Form of Preservation

Freezing is one of the oldest and safest forms of food preservation. Not surprisingly, today's frozen foods have an excellent record of safety. For example, when it comes to produce, only the highest quality fruits and vegetables are selected and then quickly washed and frozen. The result is food that is naturally delicious and safe.

Because it has been demonstrated to eliminate certain food borne contaminants, additional efforts are currently underway to utilize freezing more broadly as a food safety technology. Research suggests that variables like the temperatures and rates at which foods are frozen, storage times, and the chemical makeup of specific foods may be further investigated to enhance the safety of foods preserved by freezing. The Frozen Food Foundation[19] is committed to supporting research projects that enhance the microbiological safety of food through freezing.

The benefits to frozen foods are truly amazing, and they can stay in your home for months without going bad. I personally make sure that I always have the following frozen foods in my freezer:

---

[19] www.frozenfoodfoundation.com

> - Steam vegetable bags
> - Variety of flash frozen fish
> - Frozen blueberries (terrific anti-oxidant)
> - Frozen mangoes
> - Low fat turkey burgers (not breaded of course)
> - Salmon burgers (make sure they are gluten-free)
> - Gluten-free frozen entrees (preferably all natural or organic)
> - 90/10 beef burgers (90% lean/10% fat) or 95/5
> - Bison burgers (low fat)
> - Edamame
> - Boneless, skinless chicken breasts
> - Gluten-free macaroni & cheese
> - Value added potatoes (mashed, wedges, etc.)
> - Gluten-free bread
> - All natural frozen fruit bars
> - Sweet potato fries (make sure you read the ingredient statements—some manufacturers "dust" their fries to make them crispier)
> - Gluten-free burritos
> - Gluten-free rice medleys
> - All natural sorbets
> - Gluten-free veggie burgers
> - Gluten-free tamales (only the single digit fat per serving variety)

These are dieting staples that you'll find nearly every week in my freezer. If my day is busy beyond belief, then I set out the frozen fish that morning for later in the day or I'll put a gluten-free frozen entrée in my briefcase for a quick lunch. Nearly everything else can be microwaved, pan seared, baked, or grilled in less than twenty minutes.

Maybe that freezer lady had a point with the vacuum attachment. Now is the time for you to clear out all of those gluten stuffed foods or junk items and make way for some "frozen assets."

# Chapter Twelve

## Kitchen and Office Essentials...For A Dollar!

W elcome to the world of the dollar stores! These Stores, which have names like Dollar Tree or Dollar General, contain thousands of products that will make your gluten-free voyage an easy one. I guarantee you'll be using these items on an everyday basis, too, and, to make things even easier for you, I've compiled a list of practical tools for you that can be found in any dollar store worldwide:

## ❖ Large Re-sealable Baggies

Perfect for storing snacks throughout the day. Especially for those items that you typically buy in bulk or larger club packs at Costco and Sam's Club. Most of the meats at these stores are sold in packs of two (e.g., flank steaks, pork tenderloins, poultry breast, etc). Why not grill one for dinner and then cut the remainder into leftovers for the next day? If you prepared the item yourself with the right spices and/or gluten-free marinades, then there won't be any worry for lunch the next day. Not to mention the fact that you're having a high protein and lean protein entrée that would probably cost you $9 at a local restaurant. Do that five days a week and that's $45 per week!

## ❖ Small Re-sealable Baggies

Same as the above, but about half the size. Great for shakes or fresh fruit snacks throughout the day. These are also great for desserts. From now on, don't fret about buying large packs of dried fruits, nuts, and trail mixes. Bring them home and re-portion them for your mini-snacks throughout the day. And, if you travel quite a bit like I do, you'll make the passenger next to you on the plane jealous of your pre-planning capabilities on those long flights. Don't forget to hit the bulk fruit/nuts/snack section at your local retailer either. Those dark chocolate pieces and chips are a great dessert at the end of the meal.

## ❖ Cheese Grater

Retailers these days are finding new ways to sell excess inventory to make a profit. Many of the full service delis will wrap the small portions of unsellable cheeses and label them for individual resale. From what I have seen, most resemble the size of a small cell phone or a large hand held eraser that you used in grade school, and they only cost about a buck. Yet, if you grate a small portion of an imported cheese into an omelet or salad, you've added a million bucks of flavor and only a gram or two of fat. And, for those of you who like cheese on those leftovers, grate the whole thing and put it into one of the smaller aforementioned baggies. It microwaves well and is great in a salad.

## ❖ Chip Clips

The dollar stores usually have about five different sizes of clips to choose from that are perfect for serving leftovers. For example, there are dozens of different rice and quinoa side dishes that can be micro-waved in ninety seconds or less. I particularly like these dishes because they are vegetable and protein meal portions with just the right amount of gluten-free carbohydrates. Most of these side dishes typically serve three to four people as well. Why not wrap up what you didn't eat and add it to your meal the next day? A chip clip is hip!

### ❖ Small Plastic Containers with Lids

There are hundreds upon hundreds of every size of Tupperware-style containers imaginable at the dollar stores. They can be used to store left over grilled meats, blocks of cheese from the club stores, cut up fresh fruit, and pre-grilled vegetables. The small ones are ideal for packing a lunch on the go.

### ❖ Large Plastic Cup

You should be drinking at least 100 ounces of water on a daily basis, so having a large cup on your desk that you can fill with water is useful in fulfilling this quota.

### ❖ Calendar

It's essential to chart your course for dieting and fitness, but you don't have to buy an expensive daily planner to do it. Purchasing a dollar store calendar is an opportunity to save both time and money.

### ❖ Large Coffee/Tea Mug

Who doesn't love a nice cup of coffee or tea to start their day?

### ❖ Spatula Set

These are usually sold in sets of three at the dollar stores. A new spatula makes it easy to prepare that perfect omelet in the morning, or pan sear frozen fish. If you have a set of three, then there will most likely always be a clean one ready for use in the kitchen drawer!

## ❖ Can Opener

There are many all natural canned items that acclimate well to a gluten-free diet. Canned chicken chunks, organic beans, tuna, and turkey are prime examples, as they are all low in fat and high in protein. Make it easy to open these with one of the kitchen's most basic utensils. Buy one for home and one for work.

## ❖ Handle Scrub Brushes

I am a huge proponent of stove top sautéing and pan searing. If you always have a new set of scrub brushes for pans, it makes things SO much easier to clean up. Let's face it: one of the reasons that we don't use our stoves more often is that we feel cleaning up will be too time consuming. With today's non-stick pans and a set of scrub brushes, you'll eliminate the hours spent getting rid of stubborn grease stains! So get your pans out and start cooking more often. Besides, using your stove top really doesn't take that much longer than a microwave, and the texture of the food cooked in this fashion always seems better.

## ❖ Toothbrushes

Does this even need an explanation? So what if the dollar store has a few brand names that you've never heard of? Wouldn't you agree that brushing your teeth with an off-brand toothbrush is better than not brushing at all? Keep one at work, in your briefcase, your workout bag, and of course, at home.

## ❖ Plastic Cutting Board

No more excuses for not cutting up fresh fruit and vegetables. Plastic cutting boards clean up easily with the proper scrub brush and detergent. They can be conveniently stored in kitchen cupboards or pantry, too.

## ❖ Dental Floss

Ever have writer's block? Resist the urge to blow a few hours on Facebook! Instead, take out a piece of floss and think about what you're going to write. It's a great way to brainstorm and clean out plaque at the same time! Goodness knows how many meters of floss I have gone through just writing this book! Plus, the next time you visit the dentist, you won't have to lie about how much you floss.

## ❖ Reusable Lunch Bag

These resemble most normal shopping bags, but about 70% smaller. They can perfectly hold your plastic containers, zip lock baggies, and produce. They also offer an incentive to save money by packing your own lunch or snacks rather than dining out. I like them because they're easy to hang from my bike's handle bars when riding to and from work.

## ❖ Utensils (Plastic or Dishwasher Safe)

Plastic silverware is lightweight and easy to dispose. This means less time wasted on washing dishes and more time for immersing yourself in a gluten-free universe.

## ❖ Frozen Vegetables

I can only imagine the size of the question mark over your head right now. Yes folks, the dollar stores actually have pretty impressive frozen sections. Most frozen vegetables that are sold to them by suppliers are free of wheat and other hidden sauces (although you should watch out for flour noodles). Furthermore, most of the items are free of preservatives and additives. The next time you have a meal, be sure to include a hot side of these veggies that will only cost you pennies per ounce.

## ❖ Mustards

This dressing acts as an all natural preservative. Use it on poultry, in marinades, and even in dipping sauces. It also works well on gluten-free bread. It's time to enjoy that ham sandwich that you've gone without for so long! If you want to feel like a real savvy shopper, go look at the price tags on the gourmet mustards at your local grocery store. You just saved a fin!

## ❖ Antibacterial Soap/Hand Soap

Pick either one. With all of the snacking that you're going to be doing (fruit, nuts, etc.), cleanliness is next to godliness. According to the Center for Disease Control, washing your hands is one of the ways to limit the spread of germs.[20] Try splurging that extra dollar for a fancy soap bar. Your hands will look and smell clean, yet you won't hear your mom or grandma say, "Who used the fancy soap that's only for show?"

---

[20] http://www.cdc.gov/features/handwashing/

## ❖ Box of Thank You Cards

Once your friends, neighbors, and family know about your health issues, they will probably bend over backwards to make sure that gluten-free foods are served in their homes. A handwritten thank you is priceless, especially for the hosts or hostesses who go out of their way to accommodate you. Besides, giving thanks is actually good for your health. According to a *Wall Street Journal* article, experts claim: "Adults who frequently feel grateful have more energy, more optimism, more social connections and more happiness than those who do not." Additionally, "They earn more money, sleep more soundly, exercise more regularly, and have greater resistance to viral infections."[21] Like the advice I'm giving you? Send me a thank you card!

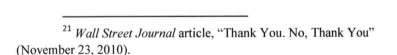

---

[21] *Wall Street Journal* article, "Thank You. No, Thank You" (November 23, 2010).

# Chapter Thirteen

## Song of the Seven Meals

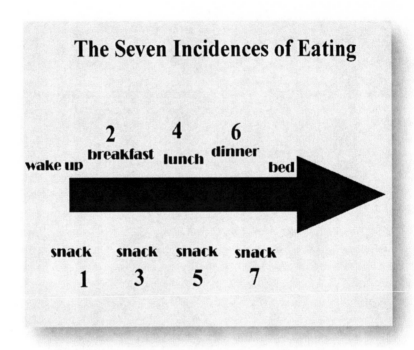

**The Seven Incidences of Eating**

For those of you like me who attended a parochial grade school, do you remember Joseph the Dreamer and his coat of many colors? It was such a famous story that Andrew Lloyd Webber created a Broadway musical about it. You could visit the book of Genesis[22] to read the gory details about flesh pecking birds, corpses hanging from trees, adultery, and of course fratricide, but let's stick with the Broadway version, as it will prove my next point.

When most people think of Joseph, they think about the myriad colors in the coat that was given to him by his father, Jacob. The garb was so beautiful that it made the other brothers extremely jealous and they needed to teach Joseph a lesson once and for all. They ripped the coat from

---

[22] "The Story of Joseph and his coat of many colors". The Holy Bible, Genesis Chapters 37-45.

his body and subsequently tossed him into a deep well to die. After giving it some thought, the brothers decided not to let their brother Joseph die. Instead, they sold him to the Ishmaelites for a handful of precious coins. They then took his coat and smeared it with lamb's blood. While Joseph was taken to his new slave quarters, the brothers returned to Jacob with the blood stained coat and created a very vivid story about how Joseph was killed, claiming it was their brother's blood on the coat. Of course, the father was crushed and a memorial was held on Joseph's behalf.

While in Egypt, Joseph, who was blessed with the gift of prognostication, immediately became renowned for interpreting dreams and giving meanings to symbols. This eventually brought him into the spotlight of the Pharaoh, who had been sleeping restlessly for quite some time thanks to a strange dream. In the first part of this dream, Pharaoh saw seven fat cows spectacularly wandering the banks of the Nile. Those fat cows were subsequently followed by seven skinny cows that devoured the fat ones. The second part of the dream revealed seven picture perfect ears of corn that were busting out of their husks and looking like a healthy harvest from heaven. Unfortunately, those golden cobs evaporated and were replaced by seven paltry husks that looked absolutely awful.

After absorbing this phenomenal description, Joseph looked Pharaoh straight in the eye and explained what the dream really meant. There would be seven years of harvest like no other. The silos, grain bags, and ancient vases would be overflowing with produce that simply were like a Ronco Christmas present that keeps on giving. Back then, Pharaoh was not only the leader of Egypt, he was like a modern day Secretary of Agriculture. Thus, Joseph's interpretation put an enormous smile onto Pharaoh's painted face, but it didn't last too long.

The look of joy was replaced with a scowl when Joseph explained that the waif-like cows and ears of corn meant that seven years of famine would follow the robust harvest. So, Joseph encouraged Pharaoh to ration the first harvest over the next fourteen years. Pharaoh most likely had no idea what a blood sugar level was back then, but the thought of moderation over a set period of time certainly made sense to him. He was so impressed that he released Joseph from prison and made him his right hand man to guide Egypt through the thick and thin of the inconsistent harvest levels.

We can learn a lot from Joseph. A consistent moderation of food throughout your day will result in an ongoing energy level that keeps your blood levels consistent. It may take a little bit of planning for you to schedule seven meal incidences throughout the day, but you don't need your own Joseph to help you through the peaks and valleys. All it takes is some sensibility and perhaps a few club packs of re-sealable plastic baggies to accomplish this important task.

Seven does seem a bit excessive, though, doesn't it? I am recommending that your seven meals be spread out from the time that you wake up until you go to bed. For most of us, that's fourteen hours of awake time. Do the math: you will be eating something every two hours.

Doing this will keep you from crashing after a meal and keep your blood sugar levels consistent. When our levels take a plunge, we get groggy and unfocused. Eventually, we'll reach for something that gives us an instant energy boost but no nutritional value. For example:

➤ Candy bars
➤ Sodas with high fructose corn syrup
➤ Energy drinks (with high fructose corn syrup or artificially sweetened)
➤ Ice cream
➤ Coffees with flavored syrups and sweeteners

However, the "Song of 7 Meals" will stabilize your energy levels throughout the day. Choose only celiac friendly foods, and you will stabilize your peaks and valleys from dawn to dusk. Additionally, celiac friendly foods actually provide more than just a boost. They are loaded with vitamins, minerals, fiber, good fats, good carbs, protein, and a variety of antioxidants. And, just like the philosophy that Joseph used to guide Egypt through several decades of highs and lows, you won't be gorging your face nor will you be starving. It makes total sense, but it does take some planning.

## Four Must-Have Supplements

### ✓ Multi-Vitamins

Take the time to visit your favorite health and nutrition store. Employees at health stores often seem like they are registered dieticians due to their amazing knowledge of what they're selling. I swear they really know that much! Discuss your current health, exercise regimen, food allergies, diets, and current prescription drugs with them. Tell them what your objective is in taking a specific multivitamin as well. With the hundreds of supplements that are on the market, they can hone in on a specific multi-vitamin that is right for you.

### ✓ All Natural Protein Powder

Based upon the "Song of the 7 Meals," an all natural protein shake can serve as one of your snacks. There is no need to reach for a sugar-soaked energy drink, candy bar, or high fructose based soda for that extra boost in your day. Protein powder that is free from preservatives, fillers, and artificial colors is a much better choice, as you can use it for making nutritious shakes. If you like working out, make sure this particular protein powder is enriched with BCAA (branch chain amino acids). If not, you can always purchase BCAA separately.

### ✓ **Branch Chain Amino Acids**

This is the name given to three of the eight essential amino acids needed to make protein, leucine, isoleucine, and valine. They are called branch chain amino acids because they have aliphatic side-chains with a carbon atom bound to more than two other carbon atoms. The combination of leucine, isoleucine, and valine make up approximately one-third of skeletal muscle in the human body. The body cannot produce BCAA on its own but only through diet or supplementation. Make sure you select products containing BCAA that aren't filled with excipients (i.e., an inactive substance used as a carrier for the active ingredients of a supplement), flavors, sweeteners, or additives of any kind. If you're into building muscle or simply toning, this supplement is an absolute must.

### ✓ **Creatine**

This has probably been the most popular body building supplement on the market for the last two decades. Although it occurs naturally in the human body, creatine is a precursor to the bio-energetic fuel creatine phosphate, which replenishes cellular ATP (adenosine triphosphate) levels during maximum intensity contractions. Supplementing with creatine can increase levels of creatine phosphate in the muscle, improving work output capacity, power, recovery, and muscle hydration. When muscles are hydrated, muscle catabolism (breakdown) is minimized.

# Chapter Fourteen

## Goodbye Ancient Pyramid ~ Hello, Meal-A-Mid!

# Meal-A-Mid (Wheat Free Pyramid)

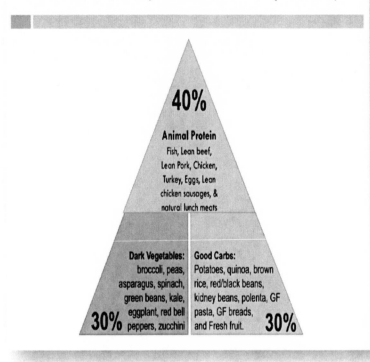

**40%**

**Animal Protein**
Fish, Lean beef,
Lean Pork, Chicken,
Turkey, Eggs, Lean
chicken sausages, &
natural lunch meats

**Dark Vegetables:**
broccoli, peas,
asparagus, spinach,
green beans, kale,
eggplant, red bell
**30%** peppers, zucchini

**Good Carbs:**
Potatoes, quinoa, brown
rice, red/black beans,
kidney beans, polenta, GF
pasta, GF breads,
and Fresh fruit. **30%**

Remember Deal-A-Meal? Richard Simmons, the popular and comical exercise and health nut personality, designed the "Deal-A-Meal" diet and exercise card game program to help obese people lose weight fast. This food program is based on the American Diabetic Association's exchange list, categorizing foods into various classes. The dieter moves cards within a wallet, from one side to another, during the day as meals are eaten. When the dieter runs out of cards, that's all the food they're allowed for the day.

Basically, the Richard Simmons Deal-a-Meal card game is a reduced calorie diet program. To attain fast weight loss, dieters are doing nothing more than consuming less food in a controlled way, by playing the card game. The plan follows the food pyramid guidelines and Richard uses exchanges such as protein, breads, and dairy. The plan also provides for a variety of choices, plus at least seven servings daily of fruits and vegetables and two servings of low-fat dairy foods.

I have to admit, Richard Simmons was on to something. Yet, his program had one fatal flaw: it was designed around the food pyramid that is full of gluten filled food. If you want to lose weight and keep the pounds off while at the same time learn to eat properly throughout the day, you must follow the Song of the 7 Meals and design each portion using what I call the Meal-A-Mid program.

The essence of the Meal-A-Mid is that 40% of your portion (or almost half the space on your plate) should be lean meat. The remaining 60% should be split between dark vegetables that are loaded with anti-oxidants and gluten-free starches. If you are a meat lover like I am, you'll be relieved to know that protein is the main stage in every one of your meals. No offense to my vegetarian readers, but your diet requires a different type of approach designed for maximum vegetable consumption. However, vegetarians can still benefit from the Meal-A-Mid philosophy, as it's designed to get *everyone* thinking about meal planning in a much simpler manner.

How does it work? There are three specific elements to every Meal-A-Mid dining experience:

- Lean animal protein
- Dark vegetables (the darker the vegetable, the higher the anti-oxidants)
- All natural starches

Seriously, THAT'S IT. Let's look at three examples of how to include these foods into your daily diet, starting with the most important meal of the day:

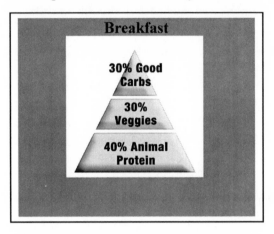

❖ 40% Animal Protein

Try one low fat chicken sausage link with a two-egg omelet! I believe that eggs are a wonderful way to start your day. They can be served any number of ways and still retain their nutritional value. Some folks like whole eggs with the yolk, while others like eggbeaters. Some people who are watching cholesterol try to stay away from the yolks, so they opt for just egg whites. If your primary care physician feels that your cholesterol level is low, then go for the yolks. They are full of nutritional benefits! If your primary care physician suggests trying to decrease your cholesterol, then opt for a liquid egg product or an egg white instead. Sam's Club, Costco, Trader Joe's, Kroger, and Wal-Mart have *huge* egg sections. Take some time to select the one that is right for you, and don't forget to get out the cheese grater and shave some imported cheeses onto your eggs. Only a little bit adds a ton of flavor.

## ❖ 30% Veggies

Make your way to the frozen food section for your veggies. There are so many blends available, including a variety of peppers, green leafed items (e.g., spinach and broccoli), mushroom blends, and Asian blends. When trying to decide what to buy, consider the store brands first. I am a huge proponent of store brands, especially the ones that are on sale. For instance, I recently had an omelet topped with an Asian blend containing water chestnuts. At Kroger, a bag of this frozen Asian blend was only eighty-eight cents, but it tasted far more like an expensive topping when mixed with my omelet! Another tasty option is the tri-colored frozen pepper blend (red, yellow, green peppers). Some retailers actually call this three blend the "stoplight," due to the colors that you would see at an intersection.

You have two preparation options for breakfast: either microwave the veggies or quickly sauté them in a separate skillet. If you sauté them, the olive oil on medium high heat makes the frozen veggies taste great. Likewise, they are filled with good fats!

Perhaps you made a salad the night before and had some left over broccoli, green pepper, red pepper, or asparagus saved in your plastic containers. You can add those to the omelet for extra nutritional value. More veggies in the morning are absolutely necessary for a healthy gluten-free lifestyle, especially when this part of the day is typically filled with carbohydrates and sugar.

## ❖ 30% Starches and Good Carbohydrates

There are many frozen and fresh carbohydrate filled foods that take one minute or less to cook in the microwave. For example, have you seen the pouches and bowls of rice, beans, and quinoa that heat up in seconds? You can buy them all in a club pack at Costco or Sam's Club. Your body needs carbs, so make sure that you add them to your plate every morning. They will account for 30% of your total meal. If you did the suggested shopping at the dollar store, you will also have an ample amount of chip clips to seal unused pouches and keep any leftovers fresh. Along with this, you can add carbohydrates by selecting gluten-free bread for toast.

Feel free to change up your breakfast anyway that you like, but make sure that you have a medley of gluten-free items to choose from. If you are following the "Song of the Seven Meals," this breakfast would actually be your second eating incidence. After you wake up, you would already have had your first Snack-A-Mid meal, but we'll talk more about that later.

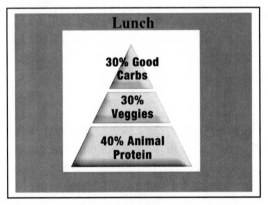

❖ **40% Animal Protein**

Examples of some good lean meats for lunch are: beef flank steaks, pork tenderloins, whole turkey breasts, trimmed pork chops, and chicken breasts. I grill a variety of fresh meat and primarily buy the "two pack" meat products offered at Costco and Sam's Club. If you save a five to six ounce portion from a "two-pack," then half of your lunch for the next day will already be planned. Not sure what a five to six ounce portion looks like? It's slightly bigger than a deck of regular-sized playing cards. Once you have readied your portion, store it in a dollar store container and leave it in the fridge!

In addition to this, there are plenty of other options that you can use to find your 40% lean meat protein requirement: all natural turkey lunch meat, frozen turkey patty, frozen salmon patty, or a lean hamburger patty, to name a few. Make sure that you shop grocery store's all natural and organic sections for items that have some sort of animal protein as 40% of the meal. If you have to look at the picture on the box to decipher the actual percentages, make sure that the protein is approximately 40% of the volume.

### ❖ 30% Veggies

This should be the easiest section of your plate to prepare, especially if you have leftovers from the night before. I like to grill a variety of veggies to include in all my lunches. Sometimes on Sunday nights, I'll grill an extremely large container for the whole week. Some of my favorites include: asparagus, green peppers, red peppers, zucchini, red onions, mushrooms, squash, and even whole heads of broccoli. Marinade them in extra virgin olive oil and a dash of your favorite spice for a great grilled salad.

Didn't have time to fire up the grill? You can always prepare a salad or take some fresh cut vegetables with you to work. Put these veggies in the microwave for a few minutes and you'll have a great side.

Remember: whatever veggies you choose to eat should constitute 30% of your overall meal.

## ❖ 30% Starches and Good Carbs

The easiest option here is to take two slices of gluten-free bread, combine them with your favorite animal protein (e.g., hamburger, turkey burger, salmon burger, etc.), and make a sandwich. Make sure that you stay away from the high fat condiments like mayonnaise. Instead, select from gluten-free mustards to add an incredible amount of flavor without any of the fat.

If you're not up for a sandwich to get your carbohydrates, look for organic brown rice bowls, quinoa packs, or all natural instant mashed potatoes to produce alternative food choices. These items can be purchased for less than a dollar per serving and can be micro-waved in about ninety seconds.

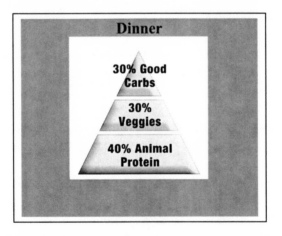

## ❖ 40% Seafood Filet

This is why my favorite animal protein shines at the dinner table: most of the frozen fish selections I buy are already portioned in five to six ounce filets, and one portion makes an excellent dinner! If you follow the "Song of the Seven Meals," you will be full after dinner, but not stuffed.

Hence, there won't be any need for turning your fish dinner into tomorrow's lunch.

You can make eating fish fun by "spicing" things up. I like to visit my local spice shop for blends that are specifically for grilled fish. Gluten-free salad dressings also make wonderful marinades for seafood. After you make your breakfast in the morning, take your favorite seafood filet out of the freezer and put it into a re-sealable baggie. Add enough salad dressing to cover the filet and put it into the refrigerator. When it's time for dinner later that evening, the filet will have been thawed and ready for the grill or a quick pan searing!

## ❖ 30% Veggies

A fresh salad is a no brainer as a side to your fish. If you don't feel like cutting up a bunch of vegetables, try frozen all natural vegetables. I like the ones that actually steam cook in their bags. They are quicker to clean up and heating them up this way sure beats having to wash a stove top steamer!

## ❖ 30% Good Carbs

Again, brown rice, potatoes, and quinoa do the trick. They are usually pre-cooked and shelf stable. Not to mention, there's something about gluten-free grains and rice that marry so well with seafood.

## Meal-A-Mid Ratios

The above three meal suggestions are only a few gluten-free examples of breakfast, lunch, and dinner. As you visualize your meals, do not discount the enormous variety of entire meals that you can prepare. All you have to do is make sure they follow the 40/30/30 ratios. Here are ten examples that follow the Meal-A-Mid formula to help you get you started:

| Animal Protein | Veggies | Good Carbs | Final Dish |
|---|---|---|---|
| 40% | 30% | 30% | 100% Delicious |
| Chicken Breast | Frozen/Fresh Veggie Medley | Gluten Free Pasta | Italian Pasta Dish |
| Three Whole Eggs | Frozen/Fresh veggie Medley | Roasted Potatoes | Breakfast Skillet |
| Pork Medallions | Bed of lettuce and veggies | Gluten Free Dinner Roll | Dinner Salad |
| Beef Cubes | Frozen Veggie Stew Blend | Small Potatoes & Beans | Hearty Beef Stew |
| Chicken Cubes/Strips | Frozen/Fresh Veggie Blend | Brown Rice | Chicken Tikka Masala |
| Salmon Fillet | Frozen/fresh Veggie Blend | Small Potato Wedges | Steamed Seafood Pouch |
| Pork Strips | Marinated Tri-Pepper Blend | Spice Black Beans | Fajitas |
| Lamb Cubes | Fresh Veggies | Quinoa & Spices | Mediterranean Kabobs |
| Ground Turkey | Roasted Veggies & Eggplant | Gluten Free Noodles | Lasagna |
| Chicken Breast Strips | Asian Veggie Blend | Brown Rice | Stir Fry |

## Meal-A-Mid Notes About Two Specific Types of Fats

The body actually needs fat to survive. It's generally accepted by nutritionists worldwide for being one of the staples of a healthy diet, too. In fact, the U.S. Department of Agriculture's 2005 Dietary Guidelines recommend that adults get 20%-35% of their calories from fats. Yet, balancing the correct ratio of good fats (unsaturated) versus bad fats (saturated) in a typical day's worth of eating can be difficult. My advice is to not get too far in over your head with your fat intake and to remember one simple rule: stay away from the VERY BAD FATS!

According to the Harvard School of Public Health, saturated and unsaturated fats are defined and discussed as follows:

## ➢ Very Bad Fats: Trans Fats

Trans fatty acids, more commonly called trans fats, are made by heating liquid vegetable oils in the presence of hydrogen gas, a process called hydrogenation. Partially hydrogenating vegetable oils makes them more stable and less likely to spoil. It also converts the oil into a solid, which makes transportation easier. Partially hydrogenated oils can withstand repeated heating without breaking down, making them ideal for frying fast foods (fully hydrogenating a vegetable oil creates a fat that acts like a saturated fat). It's no wonder that partially hydrogenated oils have been a mainstay in restaurants and the food industry. Most of the trans fats in the American diet come from commercially prepared baked goods, margarines, snack foods, and processed foods, along with French fries and other fried foods prepared in restaurants and fast food establishments.

Trans fats are worse for cholesterol levels than saturated fats because they raise bad LDL and lower good HDL. The average American eats about six grams of trans fats a day. Ideally that should be under two grams a day, or zero if possible. A new labeling law that forces food companies to list trans fats on the label should help curb the consumption of these harmful fats. Not only can consumers now see which products contain trans fats—something that wasn't easily done in the past—but many food makers are now trying to claim the high ground by using trans free oils and fats in their products.

Unsaturated fats are called good fats because they can improve blood cholesterol levels, ease inflammation, stabilize heart rhythms, and play a number of other beneficial roles. Unsaturated fats are predominantly found in foods from plants, such as vegetable oils, nuts, and seeds. They are liquids at room temperature. There are two types of unsaturated fats:

**Monounsaturated fats** are found in high concentrations in canola, peanut, olive oils, avocados, nuts such as almonds, hazelnuts, pecans, and seeds such as pumpkin and sesame seeds.

**Polyunsaturated fats** are found in high concentrations in sunflower, corn, soybean, and flaxseed oils, and also in foods such as walnuts and flax seeds. Fish (Omega 2 Fats), which are fast becoming the darling of the supplement industry, are an important type of polyunsaturated fat. The body can't make these, so they must come from food. An excellent way to get omega-3 fats is by eating fish two or three times a week. Good plant sources of omega-3 fats include chia seeds (sold as Salvia), flax seeds, walnuts, and oils such as flaxseed, canola, and soybean.

Most people don't get enough of these healthful unsaturated fats each day. No strict guidelines have been published regarding their intake either. Prudent targets are 10-25% of calories from monounsaturated fats and 8-10% of calories from polyunsaturated fats. Since no one eats by percentage of daily calories, a good rule of thumb is to choose unsaturated fats over saturated whenever possible.

Nearly all of my personal Meal-A-Mid meals are prepared with extra virgin olive oil that is full of good fat. You can use it with marinades, pre-grilled meats, and stir frys, too. There are plenty of other good fat options besides olive oil:

- Canola oil
- Peanut oil
- Peanut oil
- Avocados
- Unsalted nuts (for salad, stir frys, quinoa, etc.)
- All natural and organic cheeses

According to the former Dr. Sofiya Takh, a certified nutritional consultant with a PhD in Naturopathy and former Dr. of Science in Natural Medicine from Russia (with over thirty years of hands-on experience), there are ten reasons why you need good fats:

➢ Your body uses fat as fuel to produce energy.
➢ Your body needs cholesterol to produce almost all of your hormones, to protect blood vessels from damage, and to repair them when damaged.
➢ Your body will not be able to absorb fat soluble vitamins if you are not consuming enough fat.
➢ Contrary to popular belief, your body does not convert fat from food into fat tissue. In fact, your body can only convert carbohydrates from your food into fat tissue.
➢ Foods that are high in cholesterol and fat do not affect the cholesterol in your blood. Once again, carbohydrates are to be blamed for that.

- People who follow a fat free diet for a long period of time end up suffering from dry skin, dry hair, hair loss, low energy, feeling constant chills, and joint pain. Often their blood cholesterol level rises to such an extent that medication is needed to keep it under control. Needless to say, a fat-free diet is far from a healthy diet. What you need to do instead is eliminate the bad fats and consume the good fats. Also, combining these good fats with the right food groups is an important part of the equation that shouldn't be overlooked.
- Proteins with fats are a really good and healthy combination. So load up on those eggs (whole not just egg whites), fish, turkey, chicken and beef! Try organic eggs, as they have the correct ratio between Omega 3 and Omega 6 fatty acids. And, make sure that the poultry and beef are free range, raised without antibiotics, and not treated with hormones. By the way, lamb is your best bet as far as this goes.
- On the other hand, carbohydrates and fats are the worst combination you can have. This is what makes you gain weight, raises your cholesterol levels, and promotes arteriosclerosis, heart disease, and diabetes.
- Olive oil (which is of course a good fat) is great for salads or as a dressing combination with herbs, vinegar and spices, and is one of the best fats one can find.
- Essential Fatty Acids are…well…essential for your body! These are also the good fats your body needs for the normal functioning of the immune system, brain, heart, lungs, and liver as well as for your bones, skin, hair and nails.

The 40/30/30 Meal-A-Mid planning has worked wonders for me, but also keep in mind that I'm a male in my early 40's. Not all diet requirements are the same, so I would highly suggest letting your personal physician provide you with their nutritional recommendations.

Better yet, have them review your blood tests. There may be some instances that your doctor will recommend cutting your fat or increasing your overall fresh vegetable intake. Furthermore, your doctor may have a different opinion based upon your own personal demographics. This includes accounting for things such as your age, family history, physical activity, blood pressure, cholesterol, gender, and allergies. Your doctor will be able to read your blood results like a detailed map and help you fine tune a gluten-free lifestyle diet.

# Chapter Fifteen

## The Snack-A-Mid

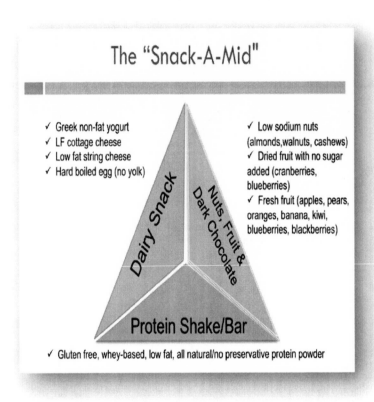

# The "Snack-A-Mid"

**Dairy Snack**
- ✓ Greek non-fat yogurt
- ✓ LF cottage cheese
- ✓ Low fat string cheese
- ✓ Hard boiled egg (no yolk)

**Nuts, Fruit & Dark Chocolate**
- ✓ Low sodium nuts (almonds, walnuts, cashews)
- ✓ Dried fruit with no sugar added (cranberries, blueberries)
- ✓ Fresh fruit (apples, pears, oranges, banana, kiwi, blueberries, blackberries)

**Protein Shake/Bar**
- ✓ Gluten free, whey-based, low fat, all natural/no preservative protein powder

I n the previous chapter, I detailed the Meal-A-Mid, but this only provided details about three of the main meal incidences per day. If you subtract these three main meals from the seven meal incidences, we have a discrepancy of four. So what does that mean? It means that you need to snack four times per day to complete the Song of the 7 Meals regimen.

I know, I know….you read somewhere that snacking is bad for you and a guaranteed way to pack on unwanted pounds, but the Song of the 7 Meals is meant to maintain your blood sugar balance throughout the day. Remember, you don't want those extremes of feast or famine. You want to snack between meals to keep from losing energy throughout the day and maintain optimum mental alertness as well. Once you get into the habit of having those four additional snacks per day, your body will tell you when it needs that extra boost of all natural energy.

I have to give credit where credit is due when it comes to snacking. My mother retired in 2000 from American Airlines after twenty-two years of service. The good news was that we could travel domestically or internationally for next to nothing. The bad news was that we weren't always guaranteed a seat or a meal on a flight. So what did we do? My mom would prepare an entire carry-on bag with fresh fruit, dried nuts, cheese, meats, and dark chocolate. We even had a few bottles of wine! If we were ever stranded in an airport (as we were many times), we had an ample amount of energy stored in those little baggies.

Do you know how many people would glare at us with jealously when we would lay out our spread of food shortly after finding out that we weren't going to be getting on a flight? To this day, I carry snacks with me everywhere I go.

So, it's time to fill in those valleys throughout your day and in between breakfast, lunch, and dinner with a wide assortment of natural food items. Keep in mind that a snack is meant to temporarily cure any hunger that you may have and isn't meant to "stuff" you until the next meal. In reality, it's your bridge in between meals, and this bridge will not only make you feel full, it will increase your blood sugar and stimulate a bit of energy for your brain.

## Quick and Easy Snack Ideas:

- ✓ Individually packaged string cheeses, and all natural cheese bites
- ✓ Snack sized Greek yogurt cups (non-fat or low-fat)
- ✓ Snack sized all natural cottage cheese cups (preferably low-fat or non-fat)
- ✓ Pre-cooked hard boiled eggs
- ✓ Almonds
- ✓ Dried cranberries
- ✓ Cashews
- ✓ Walnuts
- ✓ Dried mango (no sugar added)
- ✓ Dried apples (no sugar added)
- ✓ Unsalted pistachios
- ✓ Pre-sliced, fresh all natural apple slices
- ✓ All natural fruit cups with no added sugar
- ✓ Small sized gluten-free dark chocolate that is packed with anti-oxidants
- ✓ All natural grapefruit (no sugar added or preservatives)
- ✓ Whole oranges
- ✓ Fresh strawberries
- ✓ Fresh blackberries
- ✓ Fresh blueberries
- ✓ Mixed nuts
- ✓ Pre-sliced cucumbers with a splash of gluten-free dressing
- ✓ Pre-sliced tomatoes with a splash of gluten-free dressing
- ✓ Popcorn with no butter, just seasoning

- ✓ Baby carrots
- ✓ No sugar added pineapples
- ✓ Gluten-free snack bar
- ✓ All natural chicken strips (unbreaded of course)
- ✓ Almond butter on a piece of gluten-free bread
- ✓ Baked apple chips
- ✓ Clementines
- ✓ Small bagged salad with gluten-free dressing

If you are trying to pack on muscle, fill a large zip lock baggy with your favorite protein powder to make a protein shake. You'll always be a few scoops away from increasing muscle mass and alleviating your temporary hunger between meals. This is also a great snack to have in the morning or between lunch and dinner.

Contrary to popular belief, you should also have a snack right before going to bed. This is due to the fact that while you sleep, your body is busy repairing and building the muscle that you worked out earlier in the day. To increase overall muscle mass or tone, I always recommend a high protein/low-fat/low carbohydrate snack before bedtime. If you feel that you don't have time to prepare this, have a protein shake before hitting the hay. While you're brain is off in dreamland, the protein is feeding your muscles during the night. What a concept: it works while you sleep!

### Simple Protein Shake Ideas

*All natural protein shake with water*

*All natural protein shake with water and fresh fruit*

*All natural protein shake with water and almond butter*

*All natural protein shake made into fudgecicles in the freezer*

*All natural protein shake in Cuisinart with skim milk for a mousse-like dessert*

*All natural protein shake with ice in blender for gluten-free milkshake*

# Chapter Sixteen

## Spice Is Nice!

Picture this: some random shopping district in small town Europe, boutiques on small cobble stone streets, craftsmen and women who hand make items specifically for their customers—a seamstress, tailor, or shoe maker who makes one-of-a-kind apparel or footwear. The items made by these folks are so unique that it's rare to find a replicate anywhere in the mass-produced world market.

Don't get me wrong, you can still find personal artisans in some of the older cities like Boston and New York. But you're probably afraid of sticker shock when it comes to the price of a hand tailored suit or custom made dress. It's easy to think that custom made items are only for the ultra-wealthy and only exist in these boutique areas where the rent per square foot is more than annual tuition to a private college.

Meet your new friend the "Spice Blender" and his retail shop. Nearly every American big city and most of the mid-sized ones, too, are seeing the resurgence of spice connoisseurs who sell custom spice blends. They are usually located in old warehouse type districts and loft spaces, giving them a sense of specific cultural importance. In fact, entering these stores will make you feel like your nostrils have taken a trip around the world.

You will also see barrels of raw spice ingredients that are labeled according to the country where they were harvested. The spice ingredients are taken from these barrels and first ground to fine perfection, usually inside a room off limits to customers. Afterwards, the spices are brought to filling stations. In most cases, customers can buy empty spice bottles right off the store shelves or bring their own containers in and load up on whatever spices they want to eat. The beauty of the spice shop is that each bottle is only $4-$5. That translates to pennies per serving for a million bucks worth of flavor.

Even though 99% of all spice blends at boutique shops are gluten-free, be safe and ask the salesperson about gluten content. This is more of a problem when shopping for spices in regular retail stores. Some of the major grocery chains have gluten lurking in their blends and gravies (e.g., McCormick's homestyle, pork, and original country style gravies).

According to Food Allergy Gourmet,[23] an online company catering to consumers with food allergies, here are the items in the spice and condiment aisle that you will want to read, re-read, and then re-read again to make certain that they do not contain gluten:

> Curry
> Mustard powder
> White pepper
> Spice blends (may contain flour for consistent pouring)
> Bouillon cubes or powder
> Vanilla and other extracts
> Gravy packets
> Yeast or yeast extracts
> Broth
> Stocks (pre-made cubes or powders)
> Salad dressings
> Tomato pastes (may contain wheat)
> Vegetable starches
> Texturized vegetable protein (TVP) that's in many veggie burgers
> Vegetable shortening

---

[23] www.foodallergygourmet.com

- Artificial color
- Artificial flavorings
- Natural flavor or natural flavorings
- Demi-glaze
- Modified food starch
- Monosodium Glutamate (MSG)
- Rice syrup
- Shortening
- Smoke flavoring
- Stabilizers
- Starch

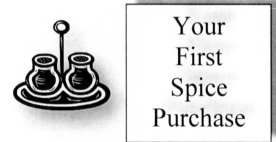

# Your First Spice Purchase

Start off small and try to target six specific spice blends for your inaugural spice boutique experience. The spice retailers have great names for the blends that they sell. At the Savory Spice Shop[24] in Denver, which is just a 10 minute bike ride from my house, simply the names of their meat blends make my mouth water!

Here are some examples of the spices I buy there:

---

[24] www.savoryspiceshop.com

### ❖ Burgers

- Jamaican Jerk Seasoning
- Table Mountain All- Purpose Seasoning
- Taco Seasoning
- Wash Park All-Purpose Seasoning

### ❖ Chicken

- Capitol Hill Seasoning
- Jamaican Jerk Seasoning
- Mt. Olympus Greek Style Seasoning
- Tan-Tan Moroccan Seasoning
- Team Sweet Mama's BBQ Chicken Rub

### ❖ Family Meals

- Family Style Fajita Seasoning (Spicy)
- Mt. Elbert All-Purpose Seasoning
- Taco Seasoning

### ❖ Pork

- Bohemian Forest European Style Rub (Salt-Free)
- Lodo Red Adobo
- Long's Peak Pork Chop Seasoning
- Park Hill Maple & Spice Pepper (Salt-Free)

### ❖ Seafood

- California Citrus Pepper (Salt-Free)
- Cajun Style Blackening Seasoning
- Cherry Creek Seafood Seasoning
- Pearl St. Plank Rub
- Tarragon Shallot Citrus Seasoning

## ❖ Steak

- Hudson Bay Beef Spice
- Mt. Massive Steak Seasoning
- Pikes Peak Butchers Rub
- Roman Pepper Steak Seasoning

You are going to be surprised what types of flavors you have been missing out on all of these years. Because of this, don't be shy about mixing and matching some of the blends into different items.

Get bold and have the spice maker blend a custom made formula just for you. Tell them what you have tried and what you did or did not like. Perhaps you're not a fan of heat or high sodium content, or would like to know what specific blends of beef spices can go well with an omelet. Once they can "put their finger" on the specific flavors you're looking for, they will develop a blend just for you. It will be custom made according to your feedback.

*Remember:*

*Even if you don't have a shop in close proximity to your home, most will ship to your house and with a 100% satisfaction guarantee.*

*Regardless of whether you have gluten issues or not, this is a great way to add flavor to any meal!*

**Spice Blends to Try:**

**Poultry specific blend for chicken breasts and turkey patties**

**Seafood specific blend (pan seared, baked, or grilled)**

**Veggie specific blends for salads and fire roasted produce**

**Egg specific blends for omelets and scrambled eggs (great on hard boiled eggs, too!)**

**Beef specific blends for grilling**

# Chapter Seventeen

## A Dozen Ways to Prepare for the Work Week

M any people find some type of excuse to keep themselves from following a strict gluten-free diet. The justifications run the whole gamut:

> ✓ "There's just not enough time in the day to do this much or type of cooking!"
> ✓ "I don't know what I'm having for dinner tonight, let alone for the rest of the week!"
> ✓ "I'm afraid that all of this food is going to spoil if I buy seven days-worth at a single time!"
> ✓ "My schedule changes too much— sometimes on an hourly basis!"
> ✓ "I am required to go out to eat with a boss or a client, which throws me off!"
> ✓ "I work so many hours that it's just easier to run out and buy something to eat!"

You would actually be surprised how easy it is to plan for an entire week using only gluten-free products. Here are my quick recommendations that add non-fattening flavor. Everything can be easily packed into a briefcase, back pack, or work out bag:

## ❖ Fire Roasted Vegetables

Both Costco and Sam's Club sell packages of yellow, green, and red bell peppers. Cut up the peppers in quarters and remove the seeds. Add one third a cup of extra virgin olive oil and a dash of your favorite spice. Marinate the peppers for at least an hour, and then roast them on the grill until they are lightly browned. When finished, store them in a refrigerated container for the rest of the week, removing only a few slices at a time. They are great in omelets, sandwiches, salads, and as a side to your favorite meat. If you like peppers to be heated, take one minute to warm them up in the microwave before eating.

## ❖ Fresh Fruit Salad

Get to know the fresh produce manager at your favorite grocery store. These are the men and women who truly know current trends with flavoring, not to mention what is on sale. When I used to live in Chicago, the local produce manager would physically take produce out of my shopping cart and tell me, "You don't want this. I will show you what came in today and what is on sale." Not once did this gentleman ever let me down. So, trust your local produce guru and let him or her suggest 3-4 pieces of produce that you can cut up on your cutting board. Then put the produce in a plastic container and you have a fruit medley for breakfast and the mid-afternoon snack. You'll also get plenty of fiber this way and a boost of all natural sugar to keep you going throughout the day.

## ❖ Salad Dressing Marinades (Gluten-Free)

Gluten-free salad dressings can give you an enormous boost of flavor. Plus, they can be used for meats. You can have a perfectly marinated fish or meat in just an hour. Just place the filet or meat in a zip-lock baggie, add a flavorful salad dressing, and let sit for at least 30 minutes. When you are ready to grill, add a few dashes of your favorite seafood or meat spice and dinner is served!

## ❖ Stock Up On Frozen Foods

I love frozen foods because they are wildly convenient! Frozen food manufacturers do a great job of pre-marinating and individually packaging single serve filets of meats and seafood. According to Packaged Facts, 2006-2010 sales of frozen foods rose 22% to reach a total value of $56 billion in 2010.[25]

## ❖ All Natural Lunch Meats

Do you remember the *Seinfeld* episode where Elaine's boss, Mr. Pitt, starts a trend by eating a snickers bar with a knife and fork? Jerry and his friends found it extremely bizarre but at the same time, perplexing. They were witnessing the birth of a new trend.

Well, plenty of my co-workers have given me a look of confusion mixed with wonder when I bring an entire package of sliced all natural meat to my office and eat it in front of them. Why? Well, I *could* bring two slices of gluten-free bread and make a sandwich, but I find it much more convenient to open the top of the package and consume it with a knife and fork just like a steak. All

---

[25] Packaged Facts. *"Frozen Foods in the U.S., 3rd Edition"* report, 2006-2010; "sales of frozen foods rose 22 percent, or about $10 billion, to reach a total value of $56 billion in 2010."

natural lunch meat is gluten-free, low in fat, and high in protein. It's also a meal all by itself.

### ❖ Low-Fat/Non-Fat Greek Yogurt

Unless you are lactose intolerant, there is absolutely no reason why you can't have at least one container of yogurt in your refrigerator, briefcase, purse, or backpack. Tons of protein and no fat, along with the fact that clean-up is so simple, is what makes yogurt taste good during all hours of the day.

### ❖ Plastic Baggies of Snacks

By now, I'm hoping that you have already hit the dollar stores and stocked up on baggies. Now is the time to put them to use. Keep them stocked and stashed in your car, desk drawer, workout bag, briefcase, and jacket pockets. I personally like to fill my baggies with almonds, walnuts, gluten-free granola, grapes, and trail mixes. Just remember to fill these baggies with gluten-free snacks!

### ❖ String Cheese

You think that string cheese is just for kids? Think again. These cheeses are all natural with over eight grams of protein and with as little as five grams of fat. They pull apart very easily and are a perfect snack to eat throughout the day.

### ❖ Green Tea Bags

Prepare a zip lock baggy with at least a dozen green tea bags in it at all times. This is a convenient way to stay hydrated with one of nature's best gluten-free beverages. In addition to this, green tea is an antioxidant that is perfect for preventing free radicals from damaging your body throughout the day.

## ❖ Dark Chocolate Bars

I have a chocolate stash in dozens of places around my house and office. Dark chocolate is full of antioxidants and it lowers blood pressure, too. However, moderation is important here. I love a small square after a meal. Oh, and make sure you eat dark chocolates only. This means NO milk chocolates. There are more anti-oxidants found in dark chocolates.

## ❖ Gluten-Free Granola Bars

Are you overwhelmed by the number of different sizes and brands of toothpaste? Well, go to your grocery store's snack bar section and you'll be just as overwhelmed. It will require some effort, but with enough research, you'll find at least half a dozen gluten-free snack bars (e.g., Kind, Bora Bora, and Lara bars). Stash the bars everywhere around you, as they are convenient, wholesome, and all natural energy providers.

## ❖ Fresh Fruit

Check the weekly circular for bananas, oranges, pears, apples, plums, and peaches. They're perfect for a grab and go.

## ❖ <u>High Protein in Small Packages</u>

These days, the club store formats have such a great variety of all natural items that are already in small cups and packages. Look for yogurts, cottage cheese, fruit cups, and protein drinks. Be sure to read the labels for any hidden gluten, and stay away from high fructose corn syrup products.

# Chapter Eighteen

No Time to Exercise?
Just Look in Front of You!
(Actually, *Don't* Look in Front
of You!)

A mericans are obsessed with television. According to TV Free America:[26]

- ✓ Percentage of Americans that watch TV while eating dinner: 66%
- ✓ Number of hours of TV watched annually in the United States: 250 Billion
- ✓ Value of that time assuming $5 per hour: $1.25 Trillion
- ✓ Number of minutes per week the average child watched television: 1,680
- ✓ Number of minutes per week the average parent spent in a meaningful conversation with their child: 3.5
- ✓ Hours per year the average American youth spends in school: 900 hours

Am I the only one that is gasping after reading this? Kids are actually spending nearly twice as much time watching TV than they are in school! Don't get me wrong folks, there are some informative and educational shows on television, but why do I suspect that the people who say they have no time to exercise are probably watching several hours of TV per day? This fact is important to consider if you have adapted a gluten-free lifestyle. Exercise is extremely important to staying gluten-free.

---

[26] TV Free America, www.turnoffyourtv.com

Imagine if you simply cut one hour of TV out of your schedule each day. Heck, twenty-two minutes of that hour is typically advertisements anyway (take it from this advertising guy, I know!). That means that you're really only missing thirty-eight minutes of a show, and there are so many things that you can do in thirty-eight minutes to make your life better.

Remember, you don't need to be sweating profusely to reap the benefits of exercise. Many fitness experts will tell you that a brisk walk is just as good for the heart as a steady high paced jog. The facts are that you will burn more calories and fat OFF of the couch than on the couch. And, you can do it in thirty-eight minutes a day or less.

**Exercise Ideas:**

**Ride on a stationary bike**

**Run on a treadmill**

**Take a stroll in your neighborhood**

**Ride your bike in your neighborhood**

**Go for a long walk with your dog**

**Lift light to moderate weights**

**Participate in a yoga class**

**Enroll in a beginner aerobics class**

**Practice on skis or a snowboard**

**Swim in a pool (swimming or a group class)**

**Walk up and down stairs**

**Walk or run in a gym**

**Practice being creative with exercising**

D e f e a t   W h e a t

# Chapter Nineteen

## Pruning the Ornamental Trees

Have you ever been to Disney World? I remember my first time as a kid catching the monorail from the parking lot to the main gate at the Magic Kingdom. As I looked out the window, I remember seeing all of the Disney characters that were shaped out of different ornamental bushes.

I learned later in life that it takes multiple years to get these perfectly manicured bushes to resemble Disney characters. The botanists are very methodical in terms of how they plan out every week of the process. It's known as a "prune-grow-prune" method, which means that the "shaper" has an idea of what the final character will ultimately look like.

For instance, the shaper may have a character with one hand up in the air and one at its side. The shaper would first need a base tree to start with that may be top-heavy to one side (e.g., an arm in the air) and bottom heavy on another side (e.g., a hand on the hip). The sculptor would then trim the bush to begin an almost snowman type base that could be shaped further down the road.

Unlike the ancient Greek and Roman sculptors who chiseled down a block of stone until it resembled a deity, the Disney botanist relied on plant growth to give more definition to the cartoon character. The bush is provided with an ample amount of time to grow back more leaves and small branches for the next round of pruning. If you have studied or read anything about shaping bonsai trees, this hobby follows nearly the same methodology. The more that this "prune-grow-prune method" is followed, the more refined the overall detail becomes.

There is an analogy here between those manicured trees and the ultimate shape of your body. If you work-out every single day with weights, you are continually pruning your body and not giving it an ample amount of rest time to grow back muscle. This is a recipe for zero muscle growth.

You only build muscle when the body begins to repair and re-grow the fibers that are broken down by using the weights. Thus, it's important to give your muscles a certain period of rest, food, water, protein, and sleep to build a better physique. You have to grow before you can prune again or you simply are going to have zero net lean muscle gains.

Admittedly, I initially did not give my body an ample amount of time to rest during workout sessions. This is what a typical workout week for me looked like in the past:

- Monday – Biceps & Triceps (Arms)
- Tuesday – Shoulders
- Wednesday – Chest
- Thursday – Legs
- Friday – Back
- Saturday- Abs
- Sunday- Rest

Are you impressed with my work-out regimen and the fact that I hit the gym 6 days a week? Don't be. It's all wrong. I didn't give my body a single day of rest in between my workout days. This is what's known as the "prune-prune-prune" method. I didn't give my muscles a chance to grow back! If the Disney botanists used the above strategy like I used to, Donald Duck would still be in the greenhouse and probably resembling one of his little ducky nephews. Rest and growth is absolutely essential to get defined muscle tone and that ripped look. Otherwise, you are that botanist that is impatient and gets the shears out nearly every single day.

For some of my readers, you probably have no desire to add muscle or get into shape. You simply want to learn the benefits of limiting your daily intake of wheat and gluten from your diet. Yet, this was the final breakthrough of my personal combat with wheat. This is what has catapulted me to the toned body that I have today.

Before my diagnosis, going to the gym was a struggle. I barely had the energy to even walk through the door of a gym, let alone lift a barbell. The gluten had also wiped out all of the villi in my lower intestines, so I couldn't absorb essential foods, nutrients, protein, and vitamins that led to muscle growth. I was in a position of a triple whammy: no energy, no ability to process protein into muscle, and no time to let my body rest before restoring any fibers broken down during the work-out process.

When I initially treated my disease and began to feel rejuvenated, I couldn't wait to get to the gym and put all of this newfound energy to work. I actually would get excited thinking about the individual exercises that I would be completing. Sometimes I would even call my work-out partner the night before and we would verbally walk through an hour's worth of weights. With this incredible surge of energy, my workout partner would push me to add more weights and more reps each week. The gross amount of lifted weight continued to go up, up, and up, much to my amazement!

While my overall intensity of workouts began to grow, so did the villi in my lower intestines. Protein became a major factor toward building muscle. I developed a voracious appetite thanks to the intense work-outs. After months of this surge in energy, I couldn't have been happier with my physical results. I was pushing some type of weight at least six days a week. Do you see this as a problem? I certainly didn't. That would change after I met a seasoned weight lifter who pointed out the error of my "prune-prune-prune" method.

This particular weight lifter was Aaron Golden, an international police advisor who worked with the U.S. State

Department and was attached to the Army 5$^{th}$ and 10$^{th}$ Group Special Forces. He had just returned to America after completing a tour of duty in Iraq, where he was the lead instructor at the Tikrit SWAT School. In addition to this, he had completed 200 patrols and combat missions while in the Middle East.

Aaron had a rugged look, broad shoulders, and a small waist that seemed to accentuate the rest of his physique. Obviously, this guy had his routine dialed in to a "T". Due to him moving in next to my house and the fact that we belonged to the same gym, we became work-out partners. I had a newfound sense of energy, and he knew dozens upon dozens of training tips for working out in a correct fashion.

In fact, the moment we began working out together and I showed him my six day a week weight lifting program, he nearly fainted! Aaron was dumbfounded at the fact that I had been doing my routine incorrectly for months. I quickly received a hard lecture from him about how I wasn't letting my body rest.

Aaron told me about how we build muscle in our sleep and that's why it is so important to get plenty of rest at night. The same was true for our bodies needing at least a day between workout sessions with weights. Only then could I hope to see my muscles grow back and become defined.

Since this conversation, I have adopted the "prune-grow-prune" method. My partner re-arranged the work-outs so we wouldn't have back-to-back weight days. The results have been more impressive than I could have ever imagined:

- Pre-celiac weight: 149 pounds
- Post gluten-free weight: 172 pounds (I gained   additional muscle!)

- Maintained a single digit body fat percentage of 9% while adding mass
- Maintained a 31 inch waist while growing, which meant I didn't have to buy new pants
- Shirts no longer fit my shoulders

No matter if you have Celiac disease or want to lose weight and look better, I am living proof that the benefits of a gluten-free diet, along with proper exercising, can help you achieve your fitness goals. Just think of yourself as that small little plant in the Disney horticultural center. The "prune-grow-prune" strategy will systematically shape your body into exactly what you want and more.

> ### Note:
>
> *I have focused on weight exercises as an example of a successful approach to working out while maintaining a gluten-free lifestyle. However, finding the best exercise regiment is a matter of first deciding how you want to look. Whether it's to have more muscle mass, greater body tonality, a combination of these two, or something else entirely, your training will deviate to achieve these different exercise goals.*

# Chapter Twenty

## Something Seems Fishy!
## (But, That's A *Good* Thing!)

W hat is it about fish oil that makes some Americans turn up their noses? Was it the putrid look on the faces of *The Little Rascals* television characters when the school marm would make them eat spoonfuls of fish oil? Or, was it the indelible vision of the nun that would historically put a student in a headlock to pour an ounce of fish oil down the ailing pupil's throat? There has to be some benefit to it…right?

Indeed, there are many benefits. According to the National Center for Complimentary and Alternative medicine:

> **Epidemiological studies done more than 30 years ago noted relatively low death rates due to cardiovascular disease in Eskimo populations with high fish consumption. Since these early studies, numerous observational and clinical trials have studied fish oil and omega-3 fatty acids for a wide variety of diseases and conditions. Overall, the evidence appears the most promising for improving cardiovascular disease risk factors. For example, studies show that increasing levels of DHA and EPA—either by eating fish or taking fish oil supplements—lowers triglycerides, slightly lowers blood pressure, may slow the progression of atherosclerosis (hardening of arteries), and may reduce the risk of heart attack, stroke, and death among people with cardiovascular disease.**

Those early studies on the Eskimos paved the way for an enormous amount of research on fish oil. Remember how we talked about good fats? One of these good fats is the Omega 3's found in white fishes. These fish are packed with protein but low in Omega 6's (i.e., the bad fats) found in red meat.

In conjunction with this, environmental contaminants that have been popularly associated with fish oils are being eliminated or removed from fish oil manufacturing. Nearly all of the fish oil manufacturers have invested a great deal of money and resources to remove environmental contaminants, such as PCB's. (i.e., Polychlorinated Biphenyl), from the fish oil manufacturing process.

PCB is a chemical that made its debut in 1929 and is known for its non-flammability, chemical stability, high boiling point, and electrical insulating properties. It has since had various other uses as well: electrical, heat transfer processes, hydraulic equipment; plasticizers in paints, plastics, rubber products, pigments, dyes, carbonless copy paper, and many other industrial applications. Unfortunately, mishandling over the years resulted in PCB's release into the environment and subsequently into vegetation and plants that were ingested by wildlife (like fish). According to the U.S. Environmental Protection Agency, "PCBs have been demonstrated to cause cancer, as well as a variety of other adverse health effects on the immune system, reproductive system, nervous system, and endocrine system."

Luckily, the domestic manufacturing of PCB's has been banned since 1979. Yet, the EPA reports that they "can still be released into the environment from poorly maintained hazardous waste sites that contain PCBs; illegal or improper dumping of PCB wastes; leaks or releases from electrical transformers containing PCBs; and disposal of PCB-containing consumer products into municipal or other landfills not designed to handle hazardous waste."

Despite being banned for over 30 years, manufacturers now employ a triple distilled process to remove PCB from their products. Ideally, you want triple distilled fish oil and whether it is or not will be clearly stated on the fish oil product label. Ask a salesperson at your favorite vitamin retailer to point out the purest form available. There are a handful of poor quality fish oils that have not been purified or triple distilled and have very high levels of mercury, PCB's, and dioxins. If you don't do your research or you shop primarily on price, you actually could be doing yourself more harm than help while consuming your fish oils on a daily basis.

The U.S. National Library of Medicine (*Natural Medicines Comprehensive Database*) listed three "classifications" when it comes to the benefits received from taking a fish oil supplement:

## Effective For:

> Lowering fats called triglycerides

## Likely Effective For:

> Preventing heart disease and heart attacks

## Possibly Effective For:

> High Blood Pressure
> Rheumatoid Arthritis
> Menstrual pain
> ADHD (Attention Deficit Hyperactivity Disorder)
> Stroke
> Weak bones
> Hardening of the arteries
> Kidney problems

- ➢ Bipolar Disorder
- ➢ Depression
- ➢ Psychosis
- ➢ Weight Loss
- ➢ Psoriasis
- ➢ High cholesterol
- ➢ Asthma
- ➢ Dry Eye Syndrome

Don't you think it makes sense to buy a few extra bottles of fish oil? It's a vital component to a healthy lifestyle. Oh, and fish oil is completely gluten-free!

# Chapter Twenty-One

TWONG!!
*(Insert Sound Effect of a Spring Here)*

> **Let Food Be Your Medicine and**
> **Medicine Be Your Food.**
>
> **-Hippocrates**

The fact that you are making emotional AND rational choices about what you eat should make you feel like a million bucks. If you follow the recommendations in this book, then you will have every reason to look in the mirror and feel good about the way you eat. I guarantee that you will look amazing on the outside and feel even better on the inside. Living gluten-free means you believe that what you eat is what you are. So let medicine be your food and food be your medicine. From the expression on your face and the healthy look of your skin, hair, and overall disposition, it will be apparent to everyone in your life that you will have changed for the better.

If you want another good book to read about food as the solution rather than pharmaceuticals, pick up a copy of *Food Is Better Medicine Than Drugs: Your Prescription for Drug Free Health*, by Patrick Holford and Jerome Burne.[27] In their book, they look at common health problems (e.g., pain/arthritis, heart, depression, diabetes, memory, hormones, digestion, breathing, infections, etc.) and compare the effectiveness of nutrition-based approaches with today's commonly used prescriptions. Likewise, there are hundreds of other books which support my personal conviction that food is one of the driving factors in overall health.

I firmly believe the gluten-free lifestyle is the antidote for feeling better.

---

[27] *Food Is Better Medicine Than Drugs: Your Prescription for Drug Free Health*, by Patrick Holford & Jerome Burne, 2006 Piatkus Books.

If you think that gluten could be wreaking havoc on your system or anyone else in your family, consult your physician immediately. However, if you want to find out for yourself or just want to experiment with the alternative lifestyle choices proposed in this book, try TWONG (**T**wo **W**eeks **O**f **N**o **G**luten) and let your body be the judge. I can see your eyes rolling right now thinking about how hard it would be to go without your favorite beer, sandwich, pasta, or bagel for a full fourteen days. Just follow the savvy shopping guidelines that I've provided. You'll find it much easier than you think.

Look at it like this: with TWONG, I'm recommending that you *remove* something from your diet and not *add* something new to it. I'm also not encouraging you to go on some new and unproven prescription diet drug. TWONG truly lies at the other end of the spectrum from an internet pill solution or dieting fads. You remove gluten from your system and make sensible decisions about what you put into your body. So give it a shot for two weeks and see if the gluten-free lifestyle is right for you. While you are trying this out, track your activity and results too. I'm positive you will find the results to be nothing short of life-changing.

Here are a few of my preparation tips prior to TWONG:

✓ **Blood Test:**

Prior to eliminating gluten from your diet, schedule a brief visit with your primary care physician. Have all your vitals tested so that you'll have a base of comparison after your first two weeks. See if your physician can check if you have Celiac disease, too. When the test comes back, sit down with your physician so he or she can explain the results. I think you'll be quite surprised by what happens in just fourteen days.

✓ **Calendar:**

Chart your course from day 1 to day 14. Pull out that daily planner/calendar you bought at the dollar store and note your daily weight, what you eat, and your fitness progress. You might start to notice your same elliptical or treadmill regimen will get a little bit easier or you are lifting more weights. You might be getting that extra rep or two that you couldn't quite attain before trying TWONG as well. Write it down.

✓ **Initial Weight:**

Record your initial weight. Your local gym will probably even have a set of calipers to test your body fat percentage. Make note of the waist line in your favorite jeans or pants. Let's face it, some 30 inch waist jeans DO fit differently than other 30 inch waist jeans. At the end of the two weeks, re-check your weight for any difference.

✓ **The Meal-A-Mid:**

Use this to build your meals. It wouldn't be a bad idea to have a copy of this prior to creating your shopping lists. Remember, TWONG is not a low carbohydrate diet. You still need to get your carbohydrates from the sources that I've listed, but it's not that difficult. As long as you continue to add side gluten-free items like quinoa, rice, and beans, you'll be fine. Build your plates around a healthy portion of lean meats and fresh vegetables and you're ready to roll.

✓ **The Meal-A-Mid:**

Use this to build your meals. It wouldn't be a bad idea to have a copy of this prior to creating your shopping lists. Remember, TWONG is not a low carbohydrate diet. You still need to get your carbohydrates from the sources that I've listed, but it's not that difficult. As long as you continue to add side gluten-free items like quinoa, rice, and beans, you'll be fine. Build your plates around a healthy portion of lean meats and fresh vegetables and you're ready to roll.

✓ **The Snack-A-Mid:**

Don't forget the Song of the 7 Meals. You need to eat seven different meals throughout the day. First visit the dairy section in the "Golden Horseshoe" of your favorite grocery store. Then make your way to the center of the store for the dried fruits, nuts, protein powder, and YES…dark chocolate!

✓ **Review Your Dollar Store Shopping List:**

Dollar stores not only make following a gluten-free lifestyle easier, they help you save money by providing you with healthy living tools that cost a buck or less.

✓ **Photographs:**

Nearly everyone has access to a camera of some kind, whether it's a cell phone, a digital camera, or a traditional film camera. Take a picture of yourself in front of the mirror. (How bare you want to get is up to you.) Many people may get discouraged by the results of their weight as told by a scale. Why not let the human eye determine how you look? At the end of two weeks, take a look at the picture and see if there is a difference. I think you'll be pleasantly surprised at what you'll see in just 14 days. You might even be re-acquainted with an abdominal muscle or two.

✓ **Eyeglasses:**

Disregard this section if you have 20/20 vision. Now, more than ever, you're going to need to read any and every label. Rather than guess what's in an item, keep your glasses with you at all times. I always have a pair on me for reading these labels. Remember that the manufacturer will always call out any allergens at the end of an ingredient statement and that's a sure way to know if something contains wheat or gluten. Other examples that are typically listed as allergens are eggs, nuts, milk, and shellfish.

# T.W.O.N.G. (Two Weeks of No Gluten Examples)

| Meal | Lean Protein (40%/plate) | Fresh Produce (30%) | Good Carbs (30% |
|---|---|---|---|
| **Breakfast** | Egg white omelet<br><br>LF Chicken Sausages<br><br>Trimmed pork chop<br><br>Lean ham<br><br>Lean steak<br><br>Greek yogurt<br><br>Turkey sausage<br><br>Pork tenderloin medallions | Fresh mango (thaw from frozen if needed)<br><br>Blueberries<br><br>Blackberries<br><br>Raspberries<br><br>Grapefruit<br><br>Apple<br><br>Pomegranate<br><br>Strawberries | Black beans<br><br>Roasted potatoes<br><br>GF Oatmeal<br><br>Breakfast quinoa (cinnamon & maple)<br><br>Seared polenta<br><br>GF bread<br><br>GF muffin<br><br>GF cereal with skim milk |
| **Lunch** | All natural lunchmeat<br><br>Boneless, skinless chicken breasts (natural if possible)<br><br>Canned all natural chicken<br><br>Frozen turkey patty<br><br>Pre-cooked chicken patties<br><br>Grilled fish tacos on corn tortillas<br><br>Leftover pork medallions (even better chilled!) | Grilled veggies with light olive oil, balsamic vinaigrette, and salt (e.g. Asparagus, Bell Peppers, Mushrooms, Zucchini, Onions)<br><br>Bagged salad (no croutons) with low fat GF dressing<br><br>Slice tomatoes<br><br>Apple slices<br><br>Tri colored peppers (julienned with GF salad dressing)<br><br>Veggie medley steam bags<br><br>Medium orange<br><br>Cold broccoli with LF GF salad dressing | Pouch rice blends (90 seconds in microwave)<br><br>Pouch quinoa blends (90 seconds in microwave)<br><br>Black beans<br><br>Brown rice bowls (microwave in minutes)<br><br>Pouch lentils (microwave in minutes)<br><br>Microwaveable edamame<br><br>GF bread with hummus<br><br>Medium baked potato (no butter or sour cream)<br><br>Corn Tortillas |
| **Dinner** | Beef flank steak | Grilled asparagus | Roasted potato wedges |

| | | | |
|---|---|---|---|
| | Pork tenderloin | Steamed broccoli | Black beans |
| | Frozen individually packed fish fillets | Grilled veggies in EVOO | Red beans |
| | | Brussell sprouts | Variety of rice blends |
| | Pork chops (fat trimmed) | Steamed peas | Mashed potatoes |
| | Grilled shrimp | Spinach | Quinoa |
| | Boneless, skinless chicken breasts | Kale | Kidney beans |
| | | Green beans | Roasted corn with hot sauce |
| | Low fat lamb burgers | Eggplant | GF bread with hummus |
| | | Zucchini | GF pasta with marinara |
| | Bison steaks | Grilled pineapple | Beet salad with goat cheese |
| | Buffalo burger | Swiss chard | Polenta |
| | Turkey breast | Bagged salad (no croutons) | Corn tortillas |
| | Lean (95/5) beef burger | | Edamame |
| | Salmon Patties (*careful here, some may contain gluten*) | Sliced tomatoes with buffalo mozzarella | |

| | | | |
|---|---|---|---|
| **Snack** | Low fat or non fat cottage cheese<br>Hard boiled egg<br>Unsalted or low salt almonds<br>Mango chunks<br>Grapefruit<br>Dried mango (no sugar added)<br>Apples slices with almond butter<br>Fresh kiwis<br>Dark chocolate<br>Fresh peach<br>All natural (no preservatives or added sugar) grapefruit wedges | | Gluten-free bar<br>Protein shake<br>Orange<br>Clementine<br>Strawberries<br>Pineapple chunks (no sugar added)<br>Low sodium mixed nut medley<br>Sunflower seeds<br>Pistachios<br>Blueberries<br>Raspberries<br>Blackberries |
| **24 hrs/7 (days/week)** | 80+ oz of water daily | | |

Are you ready to take the challenge of TWONG? It really isn't that hard once you get the swing of it. Any success in life is all about preparation and a well-thought out plan. Think about Olympic athletes that compete in front of a panel of judges, or an executive who needs to give the perfect power point presentation in front of major clients to win a huge piece of business. Or, how about the student who aces a test? What do all of these people have in common?

They all made a plan and stuck to it.

So plan to re-evaluate how you shop, how you prepare your plates, how often you snack, and when to eat. Add a cheap trip to the dollar store, and you'll have all of the essentials to follow your new lifestyle. After "Two Weeks of No Gluten," you will notice a difference both physically and mentally that will put a smile on your face and everyone around you. Guaranteed.

# Chapter Twenty-Two

## The Gluten Gladiator Guarantee

W hen Peter Parker isn't Spiderman, he's a professional photographer for the *Daily Bugle* newspaper. When Clark Kent isn't Superman, he's typically working in the newsroom at the *Daily Planet* newspaper. Well, I feel like I am a gladiator trying to destroy the many myths propagated by the food industry today that make you believe eating anything with wheat in it or gluten is good for you.

When your friendly "Gluten Gladiator" is not helping the nation to defeat gluten, I'm actually the CEO of a food development firm and brokerage company that I personally founded years ago. You probably are wondering what a food development company is, how it functions, and what types of services we provide to our clients. Allow me to elaborate for you.

My specialty right out of college was international advertising, marketing, and positioning. The agencies I initially worked for were hired by very large food clients to create new products and respective packaging that would assure an item's success in the marketplace. My creative team would spend thousands of hours on strategy and nearly an equal amount of time creating packaging that would be synonymous with a product's main beneficial attributes.

For example, something as simple as the artwork on a bottle of wine has to connect emotionally and rationally with the consumer and give them a reason to put the item in their shopping cart. More importantly, it has to exceed the expectations of the consumer in terms of taste, value, and quality. You can have the most beautiful packaging in the world that nearly jumps off of the shelf and into the consumer's cart, but it has to perform for the customer's taste buds as well.

Along with this, retail and club buyers see thousands of new food products on a yearly basis, and they have a finite amount of time to review these items. It's imperative to make sure that the product integrity is in tune with what the buyer is expecting. Months before taking a food product into a buyer's office for a sales call, my staff works directly with our client's R&D team and sales department. Once the initial formula and new product is developed, I personally work with dozens of "foodie" professionals to make sure that the formulation far exceeds their expectations. We rely on feedback from food writers, chefs, restaurant/food critics, quality assurance/quality control managers, publication editors, creative directors, packaging experts, plant managers, nutritionists, graphic artists, and many other seasoned executives.

Although the process of making changes may be daunting and take several months, we will have a final formula and respective packaging that addresses the input from all of their palates and marketing opinions. At that point, we feel fairly confident that our client's products will connect with the buyer in a positive manner. If it connects with the buyer, it most likely will also connect with the end consumer or club member as well.

This is where things get even better. At the Sam's Club corporate office in Bentonville, Arkansas, they have invested in a taste panel kitchen that rivals what I have witnessed in some of the largest food manufacturers in the world.[28] Nearly every single day, they invite any and all associates to a variety of blind tastings to gauge what additional changes need to be made to an existing product that is being evaluated by a buyer. The panelists are asked about every attribute that pertains to the integrity of the product with the exception of the packaging itself. Why do they do this in a blind manner and without a brand

---

[28] "A Taste of the The Science Behind Sam's Sales", *Connecting Northwest Arkansas*, June/July 2010 edition.

name? They do it so that the panel reflects the best quality that's available in the marketplace, and then they work on the packaging.

Believe me, when you receive the results back from the various panels, the data and subsequent recommendations are nearly 100% right on target. Additionally, the director of the taste panels will suggest specific changes that need to be made in order to proceed. Sometimes, it's literally a few extra grams of cheese that will hit the item out of the park or a few less dashes of salt that makes the product a winner. I have never been let down by their detailed analysis, and their direction for improvement has always led our items to a path of success.

In my business, it is most important to have a prized palate to decipher which items are exceptional, those that need a drastic improvement, and which ones have the best ability to connect with a consumer day in and day out. Needless to say, I have been very vocal with our buyers, industry associates, and clients with regards to my celiac diagnosis. This has resulted in my company being inundated with requests for opinions and analysis on hundreds of gluten-free products. Sometimes, a buyer will even solicit my advice on a gluten-free item that has no connection to my company whatsoever! While it's a very much appreciated feather in our cap, it demonstrates that they value our professional opinions as much as I value theirs.

In the coming months, you will be seeing the "Gluten Gladiator Guarantee" certification on selected products on our website promoting this book, as well as on the packaging of food items upholding the "Gluten Gladiator Gluten-Free" standards. I will be evaluating product integrity as both a seasoned food professional and a celiac. Due to the fact that our retail and club buyers are brutally honest with their opinions about the items we present to them, you will be getting an extremely straightforward analysis from me as well. Yet, as long as we treat those items in the same manner that our seasoned buyers treat us, you'll be getting the best facts for making an educated gluten-free purchasing decision.

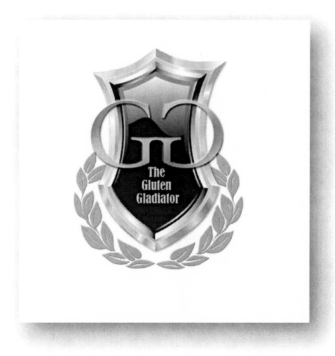

# Chapter Twenty-Three

## The Start of Something New

The last few years of my life have certainly been the difference between night and day. There is absolutely no comparison to that afternoon that I was curled up on the sidewalk in Munich to the workouts that I have every day at the gym. One thing is for sure, becoming the Gluten Gladiator has made me a new person physically and mentally. Apparently it shows, as dozens of acquaintances and even strangers have approached me to ask what my secret has been to maintaining such a healthy-looking physique. This book is my answer.

Within the first year of being diagnosed with Celiac disease, I made a commitment to at least a hundred people that I would write this book and lay out my success in an entertaining, straightforward, and fact-based fashion. If you are a celiac who has had any of the embarrassing moments that I have written about, I hope it will be comforting to know that you're not the only one out there. Perhaps you are just now connecting the dots that you may have a gluten intolerance, and this will be your handbook to begin thinking about the new way that you'll need to eat and shop from this day forward.

Regardless of who you are and why you picked up this book, I hope that you have experienced as much enlightenment while reading it as I did writing it. If you've never been gluten-free, try TWONG (Two Weeks Of No Gluten) and you too can become a Gluten Gladiator. It could be the start of something new.

## Brian Gansmann
*The Gluten Gladiator*

# List of Inherently Gluten-Free Foods

## Meats (All fresh and/or frozen without marinade and seasonings)

- Beef
- Bison
- Buffalo
- Chicken
- Duck
- Goose
- Lamb
- Pheasant
- Pork
- Quail
- Turkey
- Veal
- Venison
  Seafood:
- All un-marinated and unprocessed fish fillets
- All shell fish
  Drinks:
- All natural juices
- Coffee
- Lemonade
- Teas (unsweetened and preferably organic)
- Water

## Vegetables

- Artichokes
- Arugula
- Arrowroot
- Asparagus

- Avocado
- Beets
- Black beans
- Broccoli
- Brussels sprouts
- Cauliflower
- Cabbage
- Carrots
- Celery
- Corn
- Cucumber
- Eggplant
- Fava bean
- Garbanzo bean (chick pea)
- Garlic
- Green beans
- Kale
- Kidney beans
- Lettuce
- Mushrooms
- Okra
- Onions
- Parsley
- Parsnip
- Peas
- Peppers
- Potatoes
- Pumpkin
- Radish
- Red Beans
- Soybeans (Tofu)
- Spinach
- Squash
- Sweet potatoes
- Turnips
- Watercress

## Fruit

- Acai
- Apples
- Apricot
- Bananas
- Blackberries
- Blood oranges
- Blueberries
- Cantaloupe
- Cherry
- Clementines
- Cranberries
- Currants
- Dates
- Figs
- Grapes
- Grapefruit
- Guavas
- Honeydew melons
- Kiwis
- Kumquat
- Lemons
- Limes
- Lycee
- Mandarin
- Mangoes
- Oranges
- Papaya
- Passion fruits
- Peaches
- Pears
- Persimmons
- Pineapples
- Plantains
- Plums

- Pomegranate
- Pomelo
- Quince
- Raspberries
- Star fruit
- Strawberries
- Tamarind
- Tangerines
- Watermelons

## Nuts/Seeds

- Acorns
- Almonds
- Brazil nuts
- Cashews
- Chestnut
- Flax/Flaxseed
- Hazelnuts
- Macadamia nuts
- Marcona almonds
- Millet
- Pecans
- Pine nuts
- Pistachio
- Pumpkin seeds
- Sesame
- Sunflower seeds
- Walnuts

## Preparation Ingredients

- Brown Rice Flour
- Corn Meal
- Corn Starch
- Dasheen flour
- Pea flour
- Peanut Flour
- Potato Flour
- Potato Starch
- Rice Bran
- Rice Flour
- Sorghum
- Sweet rice flour
- Tapioca starch
- Taro flour

## Sides

- Arborio rice
- Aromatic rice
- Basmati rice
- Brown rice
- Calrose (Variety of California rice)
- Dal (Indian bean variety)
- Hominy
- Polenta
- Red rice
- Quinoa
- Wild rice

## Dairy & Eggs

- Butter
- Cheese (except for blue cheese)
- Cottage cheese

- Eggs (whole and containers of just egg whites)
- Milk (preferably skim and organic)
- Yogurt (plain, unflavored)
- 

**<u>Desserts:</u>**

- Apple sauce (organic only)
- Dark chocolate
- Fresh fruit medleys
- Fruit bars
- Gluten-free cookies (in moderation)
- Sorbets (low sugar and in moderation)
- Yogurt with fruit

# Additional Sources Used for This Book:

"Recent Advances in Celiac Disease", GUT – An international journal of gastroenterology and hepatology, DA van Heel & J West, July 2006

Jules E. Dowler Shepard, from *The First Year: Celiac Disease and Living Gluten-Free* (DaCapo Press 2008).

Centers for Disease Control and Prevention, http://www.cdc.gov/

National Institutes of Health, http://www.nih.gov/

US Food & Drug Administration, http://www.nih.gov/

National Foundation for Celiac Awareness, www.celiaccentral.org

www.fruitsandveggiesmorematters.org

www.frozenfoodfacts.com

"Frozen food forum for industry execs heats up; AFFI confirms Durant as keynote speaker, Pollster Zogby returns". Frozen Food Digest. FindArticles.com. 18 Aug, 2011.

Is total fat consumption really decreasing? Nutrition Insights. Vol. 5: USDA Center for Nutrition Policy and Promotion, 1998

"Fat and Cholesterol: Out with the bad in with the good", Harvard School of Public Health, August 2010

Mensink RP, Zock PL, Kester AD, Katan MB. Effects of dietary fatty acids and carbohydrates on the ratio of serum total to HDL cholesterol and on serum lipids and apolipoproteins: a meta-analysis of 60 controlled trials. *Am J Clin Nutr.* 2003; 77:1146-55.

Appel LJ, Sacks FM, Carey VJ, et al. Effects of protein, monounsaturated fat, and carbohydrate intake on blood pressure and serum lipids: results of the OmniHeart randomized trial. *JAMA.* 2005; 294:2455-64.

National Center for Complimentary and Alternative Medicine, http://nccam.nih.gov/

Defeat Wheat

CPSIA information can be obtained at www.ICGtesting.com
Printed in the USA
BVOW041259020112

279551BV00002B/22/P